Clinical Cases
in Dermatology

Robert A. Norman
(Series Editor)

For further volumes:
http://www.springer.com/series/10473

Robert A. Norman • William Eng
Editors

Clinical Cases in Infections and Infestations of the Skin

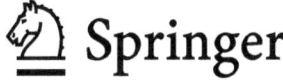 Springer

Editors
Robert A. Norman
Dermatology Healthcare
Tampa, FL
USA

William Eng
University of Central Florida
Medical School
Orlando, FL
USA

ISSN 10473
ISBN 978-3-319-14294-4   ISBN 978-3-319-14295-1   (eBook)
DOI 10.1007/978-3-319-14295-1
Springer Cham Heidelberg New York Dordrecht London

Library of Congress Control Number: 2015931544

Printed on acid-free paper

Springer is part of Springer Science+Business Media (www.springer.com)

Contents

Contributors

Editors

William Eng, MD Department of Pathology, University of Central Florida Medical School, Orlando, FL, USA

Robert A. Norman, DO Medical Director, Dermatology Healthcare, Tampa, FL, USA

Contributors

Lisa M. Diaz, DO Lake Erie College of Osteopathic Medicine, Bradenton, FL, USA

Martin J. Walsh, MS, BA Graduate Studies, USF College of Medicine, Tampa, FL, USA

Part I
Viral

Case 1
46 Year Old Black Male with Multiple Growths on Penis

William Eng and Martin J. Walsh

History and Clinical

A 46 year old black male presented with a complaint of multiple growths on his penis. He was previously diagnosed with condylomata acuminata, HIV infection and diabetes. He admitted to having numerous sexual partners and rarely used barrier contraception.

Physical Examination

The patient had three cauliflower-like lesions on his penis, one was located on the glans of the penis while the other two were found on the penis shaft. The lesion on the glans penis measured $0.8 \times 0.4 \times 0.1$ cm. The larger lesion on the penis shaft measured $1.4 \times 0.9 \times 0.6$ cm while the smaller lesion on the penis shaft measured $0.6 \times 0.3 \times 0.3$ cm. All lesions had a soft consistency and was not friable. The lesion on the glans

W. Eng, MD (✉)
Department of Pathology,
University of Central Florida Medical School, Orlando, FL, USA
e-mail: drwilliameng@yahoo.com

M.J. Walsh, MS, BA
Graduate Studies, USF College of Medicine, Tampa, FL, USA

R.A. Norman, W. Eng (eds.), *Clinical Cases in Infections and Infestations of the Skin*, Clinical Cases in Dermatology 6, DOI 10.1007/978-3-319-14295-1_1,
© Springer International Publishing Switzerland 2015

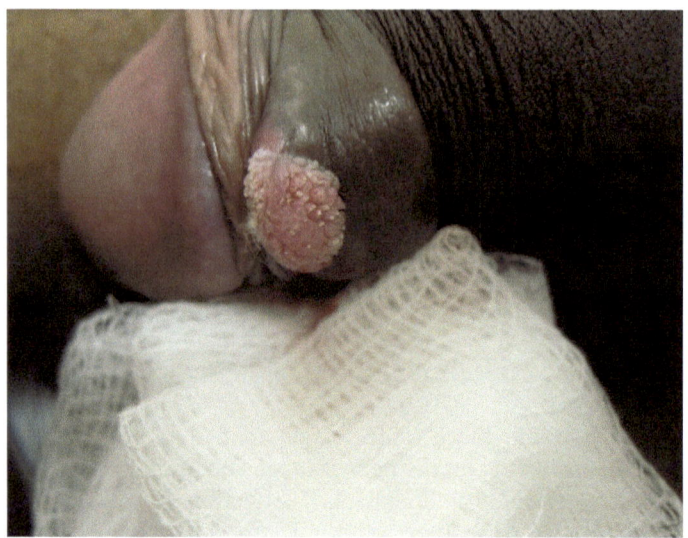

Figure 1.1 Bowenoid Papillosis arising in Condyloma acuminate

penis was pink in color while the other two lesions on the penis shaft were darker pigmented than the surrounding skin (Fig. 1.1).

Clinical Differential Diagnosis

(Multiple red-brown, pigmented papules or plaque on genital skin)

- Junctional Nevus
- Seborrheic keratosis
- Psoriasis
- Bowenoid papulosis arising adjacent to condylomata acuminata
- Condyloma lata

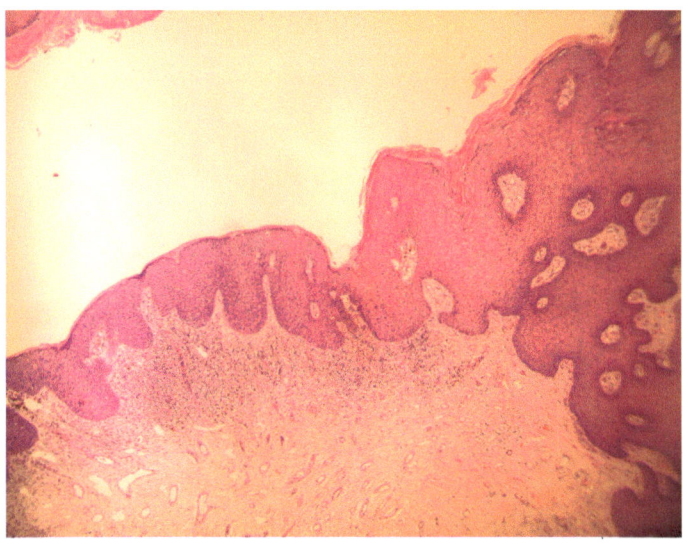

FIGURE 1.2 H&E 40×, Bowenoid papulosis on the left, while condyloma acuminata is on the right of this photo

Histopathology

Microscopically, there were two distinct areas (Fig. 1.2). In one area, the epithelium was markedly hypertrophic with an overlying low papillomatous surface pattern while the adjacent epithelium was only slightly thickened compared to the surrounding epithelium. At higher magnification, there were additional distinctive features, the area that was less hypertrophic showed marked crowding of the keratinocytes with mitotic figures seen at all levels of the epithelium, while the thicker areas showed only a few mitotic figures with extensive koilocytic changes (keratinocytes with perinuclear clearing) at the upper layers of the epithelium (Figs. 1.3 and 1.4).

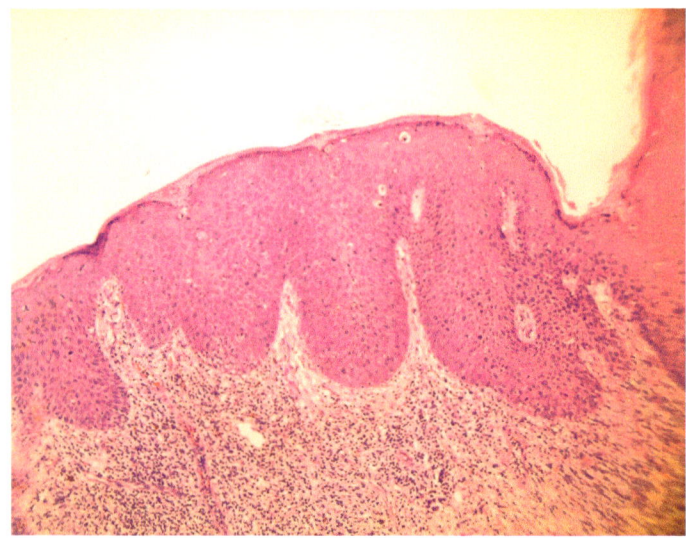

FIGURE 1.3 H&E 100×, Bowenoid papulosis showing full thickness crowded keratinocytes unlike the adjacent condyloma

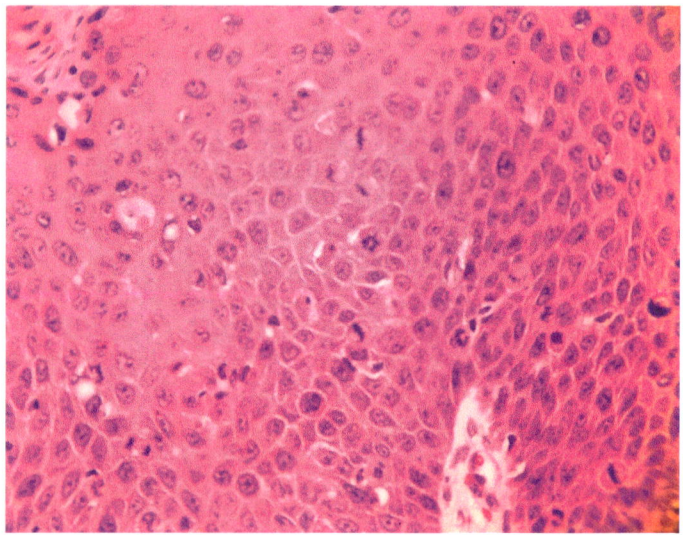

FIGURE 1.4 H&E 400×, Bowenoid papulosis showing multiple mitotic figures

Diagnosis

BOWENOID PAPULOSIS ARISING ADJACENT TO A CONDYLOMA. Bowenoid papulosis is caused by a "high risk" HPV group which includes types 16, 18 most commonly and less commonly types 31, 33, 35, 39, and 53. There is a 1–2 % risk for progression to squamous cell carcinoma so this is clinically an aggressive disease. This is considered a sexually transmitted disease, so a workup for other STDs should also be included.

While a junctional nevus can present with a clinical appearance similar to bowenoid papulosis, the microscopic examination would show nests of nevus cells. A seborrheic keratosis can both appear similar to a condyloma both on clinical examination and microscopically, however, the characteristic koilocytic changes would not be seen in a seborrheic keratosis. In cases where the distinction is critical (i.e. questionable sexual abuse), then HPV typing can be done on the fixed tissue. However, the HPV typing is performed using a cocktail, so a specific HPV is not identified, but rather a group of either "low risk" or "high risk". Psoriasis in the genital area can be deceptive clinically since the typical "silvery scales" are not seen, but instead an "inverse" pattern is found where only a sharply demarcated erythematous base is present which can mimic bowenoid papulosis. A biopsy easily resolves this issue. Whereas psoriasis presents with comb-like acanthosis and focal collections of neutrophils, these features are not found in either bowenoid papulosis or condyloma. Syphilis (Condyloma lata) has been known throughout history for its protean nature. A biopsy may show an irregular psoriasiform hyperplasia only. Establishing this diagnosis requires a high degree of clinical suspicion, a Steiner (silver) stain is helpful in revealing the spiral/corkscrew bacilli. Recently, an immunostain is also commercially available to aid in the identification of syphilis.

Treatment Options

- Surgical excision
- 5-fluorouracil
- Electrosurgery
- CO2 laser
- Neodymium:YAG laser
- Cryosurgery
- Imiquimod cream
- Topical tretinoin

Recommended Reading

Du Vivier A. Atlas of clinical dermatology. 3rd ed. London: Churchill Livingstone; 2002. p. 175.

Goldsmith LA, et al. Fitzpatrick's dermatology in general medicine. 8th ed. New York: McGraw-Hill Co; 2012. p. 1272–3.

Case 2
95 Year Old White Female with a Reddish, Nodule on Temple

William Eng and Martin J. Walsh

History and Clinical

A 95 year old white female nursing home patient presented with three lesions on her face, one of which was rapidly growing. She had a history of skin cancers, primarily squamous cell carcinomas and pre-cancers (actinic keratosis). In her youth, she spent considerable time outdoors and had multiple episodes of sun burns.

Physical Examination

On her right cheek, a hyperkeratotic growth was identified measuring 1.5 × 1.5 cm. On the left temple, a 1.5 × 1.0 cm flat, flakey erythematous area was identified. At the left forehead, a 1.0 × 1.0 cm raised erythematous lesion with indistinct borders was found (Fig. 2.1).

W. Eng, MD (✉)
Department of Pathology,
University of Central Florida Medical School, Orlando, FL, USA
e-mail: drwilliameng@yahoo.com

M.J. Walsh, MS, BA
Graduate Studies, USF College of Medicine, Tampa, FL, USA

R.A. Norman, W. Eng (eds.), *Clinical Cases in Infections and Infestations of the Skin*, Clinical Cases in Dermatology 6, DOI 10.1007/978-3-319-14295-1_2, © Springer International Publishing Switzerland 2015

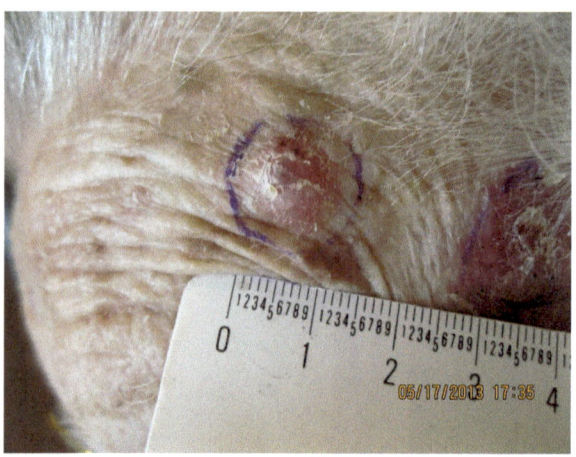

FIGURE 2.1 Merkel cell carcinoma

Clinical Differential Diagnosis

(Raised erythematous lesion on sun exposed skin)

- Squamous cell carcinoma
- Actinic keratosis
- Merkel cell carcinoma
- Lymphoma
- Angiosarcoma
- Metastasis

Histopathology

The lesion on the right cheek showed atypical nests of keratinocytes (Squamous cell carcinoma) while the left temple showed basal nests of various sizes (Basal cell carcinoma). The left forehead showed two distinct diseases. One was full thickness squamous atypia with overlying parakeratosis. The second showed irregular shaped sheets of small, round cells with scant amounts of cytoplasm (Fig. 2.2). Some areas of the tumor was dyscohesive resulting in scattered single cells in

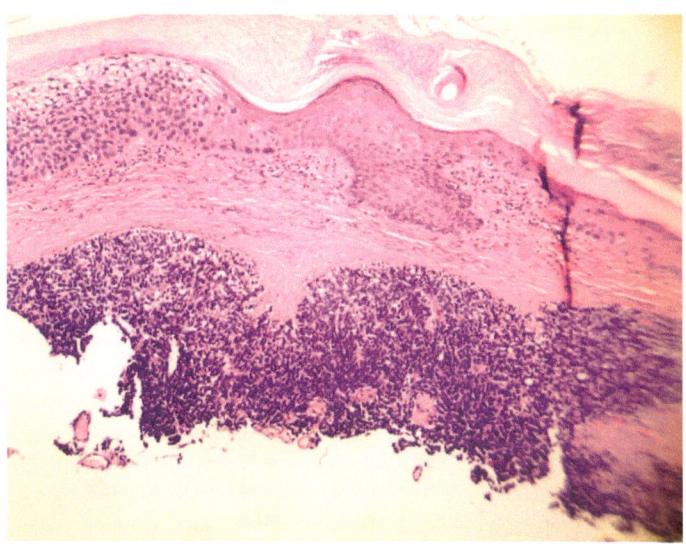

FIGURE 2.2 H&E 40×, Merkel cell carcinoma with overlying squamous cell carcinoma in situ on the left side of the epidermis

the dermis (Fig. 2.3). The nucleus showed a coarse granular (salt and pepper) pattern. These cells stained positive for cytokeratin 20 as perinuclear spots, but negative for MART (Fig. 2.4).

Diagnosis

MERKEL CELL CARCINOMA (POLYOMAVIRUS) WITH OVERLYING SQUAMOUS CELL CARCINOMA IN SITU. The left forehead lesion was diagnosed as merkel cell carcinoma. This malignant tumor is now believed to be caused by the polyomavirus. This virus is a circular, double stranded DNA virus that integrates into the human DNA. About 80 % of the Merkel cell carcinomas contains segments of the polyomavirus. Merkel cells are part of the sensory system in the skin which aids in the light touch discrimination of shapes and textures. They typically reside

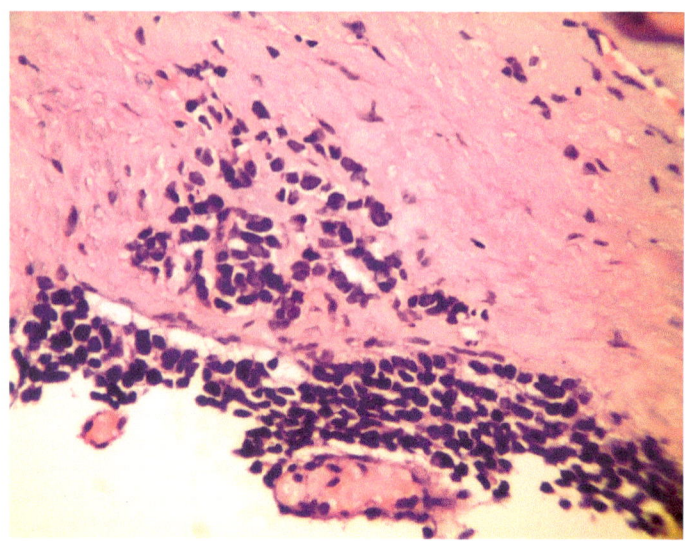

FIGURE 2.3 H&E 400× Merkel cell carcinoma. Individual, non-cohesive malignant cells are found in the dermis resembling lymphoma and other "small blue round cell tumors"

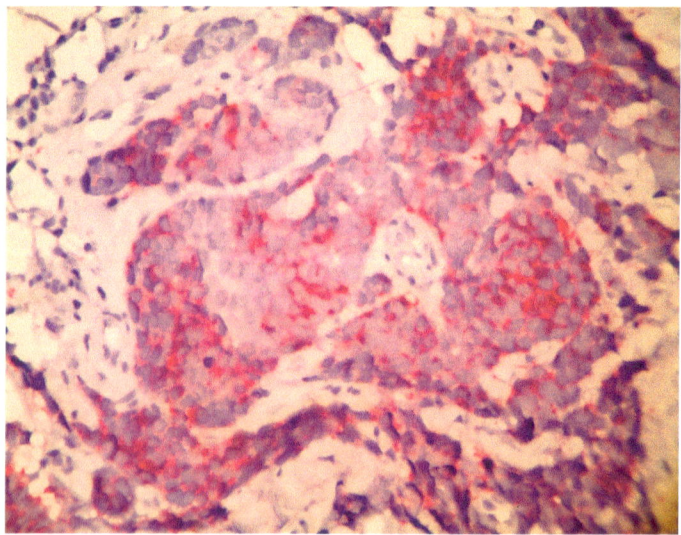

FIGURE 2.4 Cytokeratin 20, 400× Merkel cells show positive (*red*) staining in the cytoplasm

along the basal layer and connect to nerve endings and release neurosecretory granules upon stimulation (positive for chromogranin, synaptophysin, and NSE immunostains).

Squamous cell carcinoma is a strong consideration given the overlying keratotic lesion, but microscopically this invasive carcinoma contains variable amounts of cytoplasm in the dermis, and is not CK20 positive. While the slightly keratotic feature does raise the possibility of actinic keratosis, microscopically, this disease is limited to the epidermis and rarely presents as a raised lesion. Lymphoma is an excellent consideration in the differential clinically, however, more than one lesion would be expected. Microscopically, lymphoma would also have to be ruled out given the microscopic pattern and this can be done by immunostaining. Lymphoma would be positive for LCA, but negative for CK20. Angiosarcoma can easily be excluded by microscopic examination. It has large, irregular cells with vascular channels. If there is doubt, then a CD34, Factor 8, or vWB stain can be done to highlight its vascular origin. This tumor is negative for CK20. A metastatic neuroendocrine tumor is the most difficult tumor to distinguish, Both the clinical and histiologically appearance would be the same as well as both having CK20 positive staining. Whereas Merkel cell carcinoma (skin primary) is negative for TTF-1, a metastatic neuroendocrine tumor from the lung would be positive in the vast majority of cases.

Prognosis and Lymph Nodes

A study by Memorial Sloan-Kettering found that the 5 year survival rate was 75, 59 and 25 % for localized, regional, and distant disease, respectively. Sentinel lymph node biopsy, if positive, does appear to be helpful in determining adjuvant therapy.

The current treatment algorithm is not based on randomized control trials due to the fact that the tumor is so rare. Complete excision, whether with Mohs surgery or elliptical excision is paramount. However, recurrence is still common. In one study with 5 mm surgical margins, there was 100 %

recurrence. Another study showed recurrence of 49 % despite 2.5 cm or greater surgical margins. Chemotherapy (Etoposide and Cisplatin/carboplatin) portends higher mortality in some studies. However, the tumor is generally sensitive to radiation therapy.

Recommended Reading

Goldsmith LA, et al. Fitzpatrick's dermatology in general medicine. 8th ed. New York: McGraw-Hill Co; 2012. p. 1362–70.

Case 3
40 Year Old White Female with an Itchy, Widespread Rash

William Eng and Martin J. Walsh

History and Clinical

A 40-year-old white female presented with erythematous plaques with whitish streaks that had spread throughout her body. On the first occurrence of these rashes, she visited an emergency room where she was given glucocorticoid injections. The patient was instructed to see her primary care physician, where she was given a topical steroid ointment and oral steroid tablets. The patient had stopped taking the steroid tablets due to weight gain and increased fluid retention, even though they were resolving the skin lesions. The physician diagnosed the condition as psoriasis although no biopsy was done. The patient also had a history of diabetes and had noted that heat and stress made her skin lesions worse. A recent laboratory test revealed that she had elevated hepatitis C antibodies.

‾‾‾‾‾‾‾‾

W. Eng, MD (✉)
Department of Pathology,
University of Central Florida Medical School,
Orlando, FL, USA
e-mail: drwilliameng@yahoo.com

M.J. Walsh, MS, BA
Graduate Studies, USF College of Medicine, Tampa, FL, USA

R.A. Norman, W. Eng (eds.), *Clinical Cases in Infections*   15
and Infestations of the Skin, Clinical Cases in Dermatology 6,
DOI 10.1007/978-3-319-14295-1_3,
© Springer International Publishing Switzerland 2015

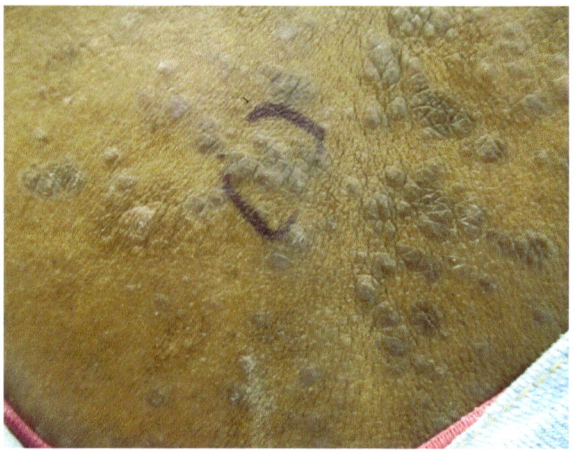

FIGURE 3.1 Lichen Planus

Physical Examination

The patient upon examination showed signs of pruritus and ichthyosis where the hypo- pigmented lesions were present. A shave biopsy was performed on a lesion located on the inferior medial portion of the mid-back (Fig. 3.1), which measured $1.0 \times 0.8 \times 0.1$ cm.

Clinical Differential Diagnosis

- Drug eruption
- Lichen Planus secondary to Hepatitis C infection
- Psoriasis
- Tinea
- Contact dermatitis

Histopathology

Sections showed a band-like infiltrate of lymphocytes along the epidermal/dermal junction. The junction showed "sawtooth" like changes. Focal wedge shaped hypergranulosis was seen (Fig. 3.2) Period Acid-Schiff stain tested negative for fungus.

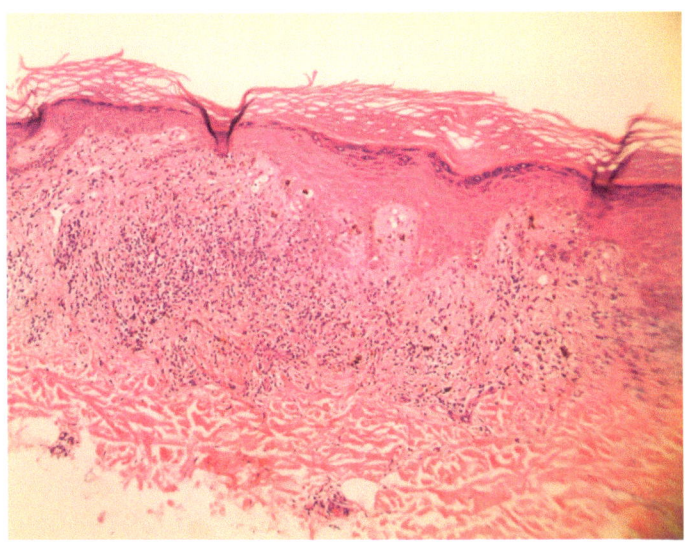

FIGURE 3.2 H&E 100×, Lichen planus eruption secondary to Hepatitis C infection

Diagnosis

LICHEN PLANUS SECONDARY TO HEPATITIS C INFECTION. Hepatitis C is found in between 16 and 29 % of patients with lichen planus, and believed to be a trigger event. There is also an association with other liver diseases such as autoimmune chronic active hepatitis, primary biliary cirrhosis, and post viral chronic active hepatitis. D-penicillamine is known to exacerbate lichen planus. Lichen planus has been given the nickname "4P" to describe its clinical appearance, Pigmented, Purpuric, Pruritic, Plaques.

A drug eruption can have a variety of patterns; perivascular, lichenoid, psoriasiform, and interface. A clue to drug etiology is the presence of a few eosinophils combined with a clinical history of an eruption shortly after ingestion of the offending drug. A benign lichenoid keratosis is usually a solitary lesion and rarely contains eosinophils. Other lichenoid processes like erythema multiforme, TEN, Graft vs Host disease all have distinctive clinical presentations. Erythema multiforme has a target-like pattern. Graft vs host has a history of a transplant such as a bone marrow transplant. Psoriasis can have a similar clinical appearance, however, the distinction is readily made microscopically. Psoriasis has a characteristic comb-like acanthuses with collections of neutrophils (Pautriers micro abscess). The scaly texture can raise the differential of tinea clinically, but microscopic examination only shows a sparse perivascular lymphocytic infiltrate with PAS positive staining fungal hyphae. A contact dermatitis could be considered microscopically, however, contact dermatitis is typically confluent with sharply demarcated borders.

Treatment Options

- Steroids (topical and systemic)
- Topical retinoids
- Tacrolimus
- Pimecrolimus
- Cyclosporine
- Phototherapy

Recommended Reading

Goldsmith LA et al. Fitzpatrick's dermatology in general medicine. 8th ed. New York: McGraw-Hill Co; 2012. p. 296–316.

Case 4
29 Year Old White Female with Grouped Blisters on Left Thigh

William Eng and Martin J. Walsh

History and Clinical

A 29-year-old white female prostitute presented with a group of vesicular lesions on her interior left thigh.

Physical Examination

The patient revealed grouped and localized vesicular lesions that were surrounded by erythema. The lesion had increased in size and number of vesicles. The vesicles were easily ruptured which revealed a raw, tender base. The blister fluid was clear to yellowish with a watery consistency (Fig. 4.1).

W. Eng, MD (✉)
Department of Pathology, University of Central Florida
Medical School, Orlando, FL, USA
e-mail: drwilliameng@yahoo.com

M.J. Walsh, MS, BA
Graduate Studies, USF College of Medicine, Tampa, FL, USA

R.A. Norman, W. Eng (eds.), *Clinical Cases in Infections and Infestations of the Skin*, Clinical Cases in Dermatology 6, DOI 10.1007/978-3-319-14295-1_4, © Springer International Publishing Switzerland 2015

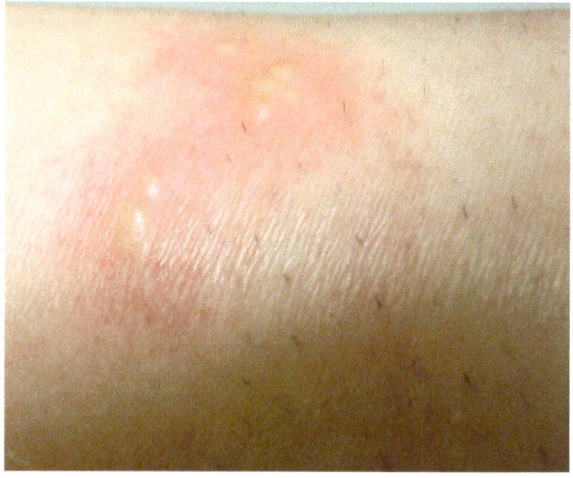

FIGURE 4.1 Herpes eruption on the interior portion of the left thigh

Clinical Differential Diagnosis

- Drug eruption
- Bullous pemphigoid
- Pemphigus vulgaris
- Linear IgA disease
- Herpes simplex viral infection (type 2)
- Bullous dermatophytosis
- Bullous lichen planus

Histopathology

A shave biopsy was performed which measured $0.8 \times 0.4 \times 0.2$ cm. Sections showed a fluid filled vesicle marked with extensive acantholysis and necrosis of the keratinocytes (Fig. 4.2) Scattered keratinocytes showed "nuclear molding" while other areas showed "nuclear margination" (Fig. 4.3).

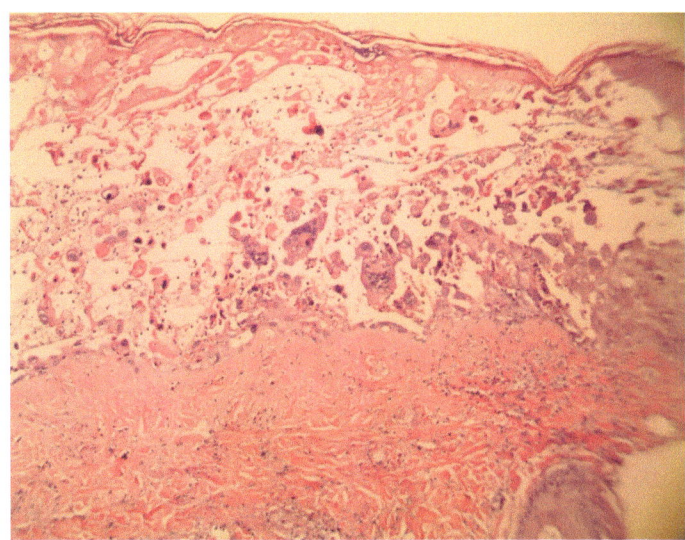

FIGURE 4.2 H&E 100×. Herpes simplex Type 2, acantholysis and necrosis of keratinocytes

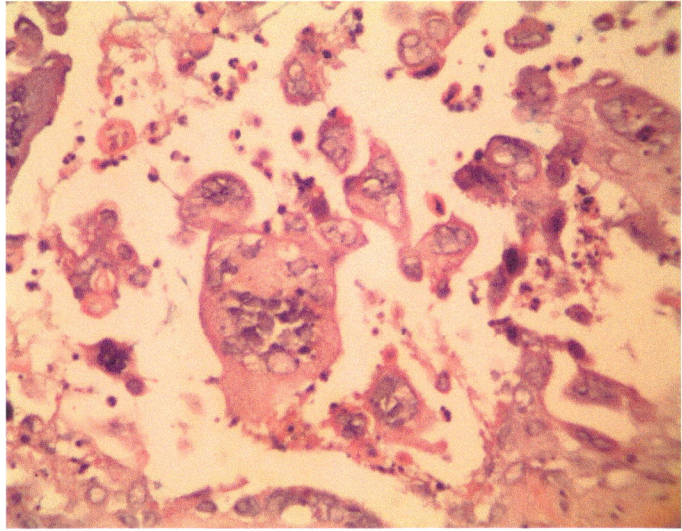

FIGURE 4.3 H&E 400× Herpes simplex Type 2, showing multinuclear keratinocytes with nuclear margination where the nuclear material is denser along the nucleus edge while the central area of the nucleus shows clearing

Diagnosis

HERPES SIMPLEX VIRAL INFECTION (TYPE 2) This patient most likely acquired this viral infection through sexual contact. Serological studies showed increased IgG titers which supports a recurrent lesion. HSV Type 1 infection is commonly known as "cold sores" and found around the mouth. Both are double stranded DNA viruses. After the initial infection, the virus becomes incorporated with the nerve of the host's DNA. Decreases in cellular immunity can trigger recurrences of infection.

Drug eruptions, particularly with interface changes, are prone to separation of the epidermis from the underlying dermis. However microscopically, they do not have severe epidermal necrosis, nor the acantholysis, nor the multinucleated keratinocytes found in herpes. The immunobullous diseases such as bullous pemphigoid and EBA shows numerous eosinophils along with a sub epidermal blister. Direct immunofluorescence will show a fine, linear junctional deposits of IgG and C3. Pemphigus vulgaris shows a supra basal blister with intercellular deposits of IgG which gives a fishnet-like appearance by direct immunofluorescence. Linear IgA disease can present as a "necklace" of blisters clinically. Direct immunofluorescence generates a linear deposit of IgA along the junction.

Treatment Options

- Acyclovir
- Valacyclovir

Recommended Reading

Goldsmith LA et al. Fitzpatrick's dermatology in general medicine. 8th ed. New York: McGraw-Hill Co; 2012. p. 2367–82.

Case 5
70 Year Old White Male with Grouped Blisters on Right Lower Leg

William Eng and Lisa M. Diaz

History and Clinical

A 70-year-old male presented with a painful, itchy rash. The rash began with an itchy sensation which then transformed into blisters that were easily breakable. The patient was a long term resident at a local nursing home. The patient was also allergic to Zocor and Fluvastatin.

Physical Examination

These lesions on his right lower extremity showed a follicular-centric rash and were confined to a dermatome pattern (Fig. 5.1). Closer examination showed vesicular lesions on an erythematous base (Fig. 5.2). When the vesicles break, it resolved with hyper pigmentation (Fig. 5.3).

W. Eng, MD (✉)
Department of Pathology, University of Central Florida Medical School, Orlando, FL, USA
e-mail: drwilliameng@yahoo.com

L.M. Diaz, DO
Lake Erie College of Osteopathic Medicine, Bradenton, FL, USA

R.A. Norman, W. Eng (eds.), *Clinical Cases in Infections and Infestations of the Skin*, Clinical Cases in Dermatology 6, DOI 10.1007/978-3-319-14295-1_5,
© Springer International Publishing Switzerland 2015

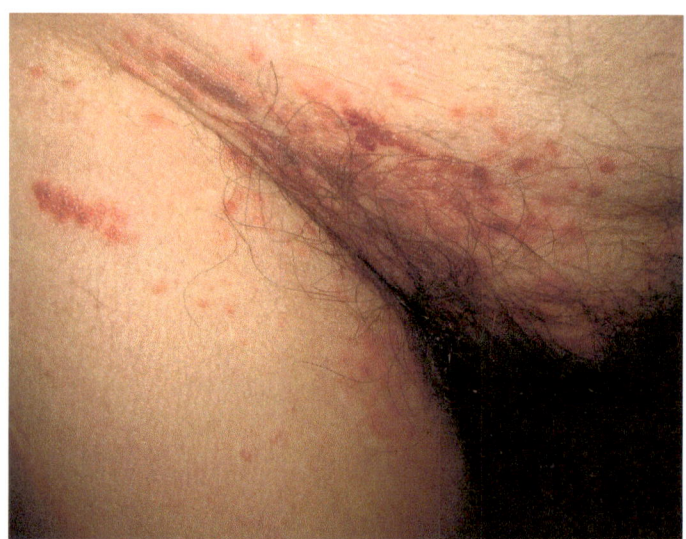

FIGURE 5.1 Herpes Zoster, note the dermatome distribution

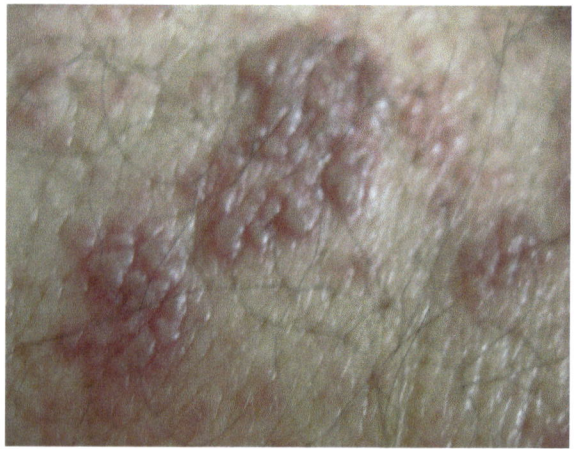

FIGURE 5.2 Herpes zoster, vesicles themselves appear the same as herpes simplex

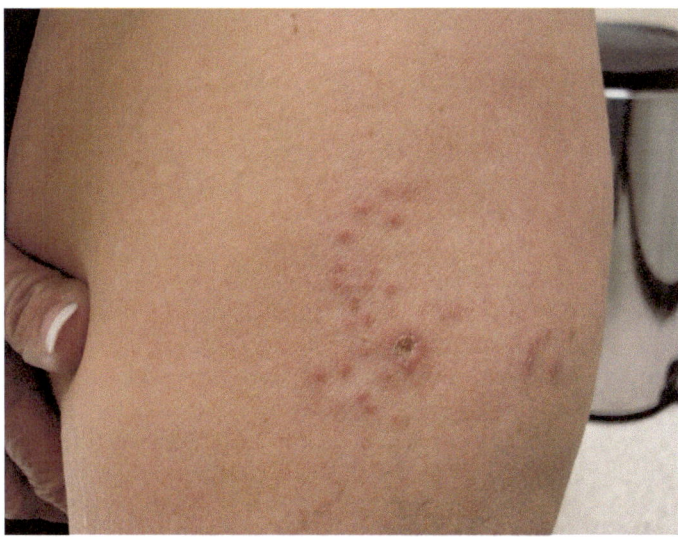

FIGURE 5.3 Herpes Zoster, note the grouped vesicles in this resolved lesion

Clinical Differential Diagnosis

- Drug eruption
- Herpes Zoster with follicular involvement
- Bullous pemphigoid
- Stasis blister

Histopathology

A shave biopsy was taken from the right lower leg and it measured $0.7 \times 0.5 \times 0.1$ cm. Sections showed extensive acantholysis and necrosis of the keratinocytes. Nuclear molding and margination were also noted within the follicular epithelium as well.

Diagnosis

HERPES ZOSTER WITH FOLLICULAR INVOLVEMENT. This lesion represents reactivation of varicella (chicken pox). After the initial infection, the virus is integrated within the nerve nucleus, only to re-emerge when cell mediate immunity is weakened. Natural aging, those over 50 years old face a slow decline in the cellular immunity so the risk of herpes zoster rises over time. Pain is the most common complication (post-herpetic neuralgia). Folliculitis is defined as inflammation of the hair follicle. When herpes simplex virus or varicella zoster virus infects the hair follicle, the result is herpes folliculitis (Fig. 5.4). This is a rare diagnosis, there are less than 30 reported cases of herpes folliculitis in the literature. It is difficult for dermatologists to determine that a virus is the cause of the folliculitis based solely on the clinical presentation. Usually the diagnosis is not made until treatments for bacte-

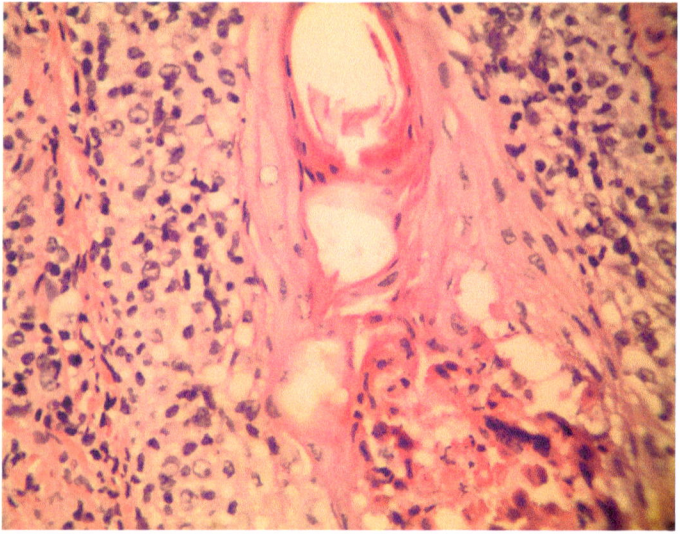

Fig. 5.4 H&E 400×, Herpes folliculitis, HSV changes are found within the follicular epithelium

rial and fungal folliculitis have failed. At that point, the work up progresses until the viral cause is exposed.

A typical cutaneous herpetic infection presents as grouped vesicles on an erythematous base. These vesicles evolve into pustules that eventually rupture and form an overlying crust. The lesions can be pruritic and painful. Herpes folliculitis, however, does not present as a typical herpetic infection. Rather it assumes the guise of a characteristic folliculitis with folliculocentric papules or pustules on an erythematous base. In the past, herpes folliculitis was thought to be caused by the herpes simplex virus (HSV-1 or HSV-2). Recent literature argues that herpes folliculitis is more common in patients who have a varicella zoster virus (VZV) infection than a HSV infection. Using polymerase chain reaction studies for specific DNA, a study by Boer et al. demonstrated that out of 21 subjects diagnosed with herpes folliculitis, 17 tested positive for VZV, four were positive for HSV-1, and none tested positive for HSV-2.

Under the microscope, herpes folliculitis may be confused with lymphoma. One study demonstrated a case of "pseudo-lymphoma" in which the diagnosis of lymphoma was made incorrectly. The pathologist was confused by the prominent lymphoid infiltrate laden with CD-30 positive cells that is so similar to the histological presentation of lymphoma. As mentioned earlier, the diagnosis of herpes folliculitis is generally not even considered until management for both bacterial and fungal folliculitis fail. At that point, a more involved work up can be performed which would include a PCR study for HSV-1, HSV-2 or VZV DNA.

A drug eruption is common among the elderly and the presence of eosinophils along with the temporal proximity of the exposure to the offending drug is helpful in establishing the diagnosis. Bullous pemphigoid is characterized by a marked eosinophilic infiltrate with a subepidermal blister. Confirmation is done by observing deposits of fine granular IgG and C3 with direct immunofluorescence testing. A stasis blister is also common in elderly patients with a declining cardiovascular function. The blister itself elicits minimal inflammation, but markedly thickened superficial vessels are found often with pigment incontinence.

Treatment Options

Once the correct diagnosis has been made, the literature reports good outcomes with valacyclovir and acyclovir. In one study by Jang and Kim, an antihistamine was added to the regimen of acyclovir with a good result and improvement of pruritus. An interesting study published by Bello and Burgos described a relapsing non-Hodgkin lymphoma patient who presented with extensive follicular lesions for 1 month. After biopsy, the pathology was consistent with necrotizing herpes folliculitis. It was treated successfully valacyclovir with full remission of the lesions.

- Antivirals, Famvir 500 mg four times daily oral tablets and Triamcinolone 0.1 % twice daily topical cream.
- Pain management

    Lidocaine patch
    Capsaicin
    Gabapentin
    Pregabalin
    Opioids
    Tricyclic antidepressants

Prevention

Due to the highly contagious nature of cutaneous viral infections, it is recommended that males with beards avoid shaving over or near cold sores. Otherwise, good hygiene is encouraged. In summary, in cases of recurrent or recalcitrant folliculitis, the dermatologist is encouraged to consider herpes folliculitis in the differential. The zoster vaccine (Zostavax) is a live attenuated virus recommended for patients over 50 years old. In the clinical trial, the vaccine reduced the incidence of zoster outbreak by 69 % in the 50–59 year old age group. However, the effectiveness decreased to 18 % in the over 80 year old age group. The overall reduction of zoster outbreak in this vaccine study was 51 %.

Recommended Reading

Al-Dhafiri SA, Molinari R. Herpetic folliculitis. J Cutan Med Surg. 2002;6(1):19–22.

Bello CC, Burgos SC, Cardenas CD, Gonzalez SB. Necrotizing herpes folliculitis: report of one case. Rev Med Chil. 2012;140(12): 1589–92.

Boer A, Herder N, Winter K, Falk T. Herpes folliculitis: clinical, histopathological, and molecular pathologic observances. Br J Dermatol. 2006;154(4):743–6.

Foti C, Calvario A, d'Ovidio R, et al. Recalcitrant scalp folliculitis: a possible role of herpes simplex virus type 2. New Microbiol. 2005;28(2):157–9.

Jang KA, Kim SH, Choi JH, et al. Viral folliculitis on the face. Br J Dermatol. 2000;142(3):555–9.

Merek. Full Prescribing Information for Zostavax, February 2014.

Wayne G. Herpes simplex virus infections. In: Calonje E, Brenn T, Lazar A, editors. McKee's pathology of the skin. 4th ed. Waltham MA: Elsevier Limited; 2012.

Case 6
2 Year Old White Female with Multiple, Small, Smooth Dome-Like Papules on Left Cheek

William Eng and Martin J. Walsh

History and Clinical

A 2-year-old white female presented with a solitary growth on her left facial cheek. The patient's mother witnessed her scratching her face, arms, and legs.

Physical Examination

The examination showed a pink-whitish smooth dome-shaped papule measuring about 2 mm in diameter (Fig. 6.1). The patient showed mild erythema with fine scaling at the periphery of this lesion. Occasional pinpoint areas of bleeding were also noted in areas of excoriation.

W. Eng, MD (✉)
Department of Pathology,
University of Central Florida Medical School, Orlando, FL, USA
e-mail: drwilliameng@yahoo.com

M.J. Walsh, MS, BA
Graduate Studies,
USF College of Medicine, Tampa, FL, USA

R.A. Norman, W. Eng (eds.), *Clinical Cases in Infections and Infestations of the Skin*, Clinical Cases in Dermatology 6, DOI 10.1007/978-3-319-14295-1_6, © Springer International Publishing Switzerland 2015

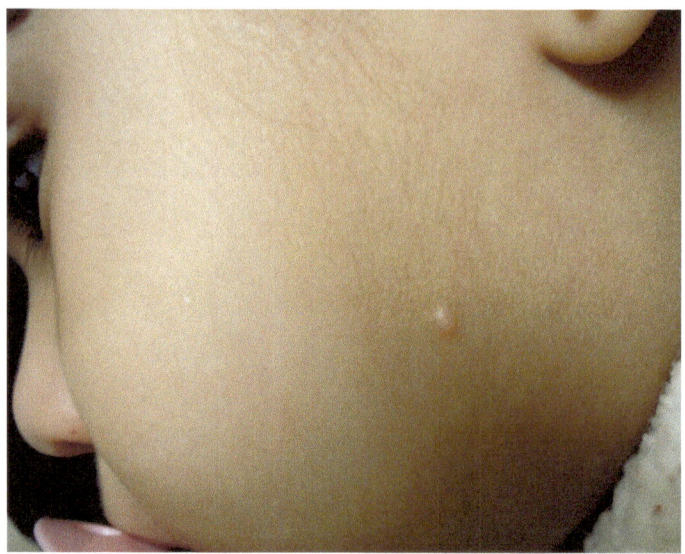

FIGURE 6.1 Molloscum contagiosum

Clinical Differential Diagnosis

- Milia cyst
- Pyogenic granuloma
- Sebaceous hyperplasia
- Molloscum contagiosum
- Keratoacanthoma
- Papular granuloma annulare
- Fungal infections

Histopathology

The biopsy specimen from the left cheek measured $0.1 \times 0.1 \times 0.1$ cm. Microscopic sections showed a lobular pro-liferation of keratinocytes. Some keratinocytes were enlarged and have a foamy vacuolated cytoplasm in the center of the lesion. Other keratinocytes were lost their nucleus and were brightly eosinophilic (Fig. 6.2).

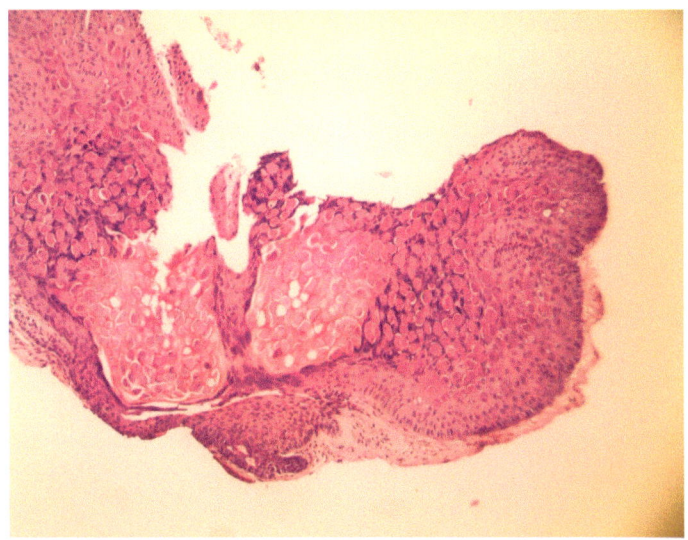

FIGURE 6.2 H&E 40×, Molloscum contagiosum, large round eosinophilic foamy, globules are found within the cytoplasm of keratinocytes

Diagnosis

MOLLOSCUM CONTAGIOSUM ARISING IN A BACKGROUND OF ATOPIC DERMATITIS. Molloscum belongs to the Pox family of viruses which often affects children. The patient's skin condition was diagnosed as atopic dermatitis which places the patient at an increased risk for contracting molloscum virus.

A milia cyst has a similar clinical appearance to molloscum, but the microscopic examination easily distinguishes them. The milia cyst is lined by a thin layer of stratified squamous epithelium and contains loose cornified material centrally. Pyogenic granuloma (PG) can have a similar shape to molloscum, but it is typically reddish in color. Microscopically, PG have multiple groups of small vessels. Another small papule that is commonly found on the face is sebaceous hyperplasia.

Upon closer examination, one could see a faint lobulated pattern with a yellowish hue. Microscopically, sebaceous hyperplasia shows markedly enlarged sebaceous lobules without atypia. Keratoacanthomas also present as a dome-shaped lesion, but it is typically much larger than Molloscum (7–10 mm vs 2–3 mm). Similar to Molloscum, it can have a central crater as well. Keratoacanthomas are typically found in the elderly population on sun damaged skin. The papular variant of granuloma annulare typically presents as small round groups, although individually, it can look similar to Molloscum. In this disease, histiocytes are seen engulfing collagen bundles. Fungal infections can have the appearance of small domed papules, but special stains (**PAS or GMS**) or fungal cultures can be utilized to identify the causative organism.

Treatment Options

- Tacrolimus 0.03 % topical ointment for the eczema
- Cantharidin
- Curettage
- Cryotherapy
- Imiquimod

Recommended Reading

Goldsmith LA et al. Fitzpatrick's dermatology in general medicine. 8th ed. New York: McGraw-Hill Co; 2012. p. 2417–20.

Case 7
6 Year Old White Male with Recurrent Brownish Patches Around Mouth

William Eng and Martin J. Walsh

History and Clinical

A 6-year-old male presented with a recurrent lesion around the mouth. These lesions were frozen with liquid nitrogen therapy at his previous visit but the lesions still persisted. The patient was using Desonide 0.05 % topical cream.

Physical Examination

The patient showed signs of normal mood, affect, and alertness. The patient was observed to have multiple brown to tan macules primary around his mouth (Fig. 7.1).

W. Eng, MD (✉)
Department of Pathology, University of Central Florida Medical School, Orlando, FL, USA
e-mail: drwilliameng@yahoo.com

M.J. Walsh, MS, BA
Graduate Studies, USF College of Medicine, Tampa, FL, USA

R.A. Norman, W. Eng (eds.), *Clinical Cases in Infections and Infestations of the Skin*, Clinical Cases in Dermatology 6, DOI 10.1007/978-3-319-14295-1_7,
© Springer International Publishing Switzerland 2015

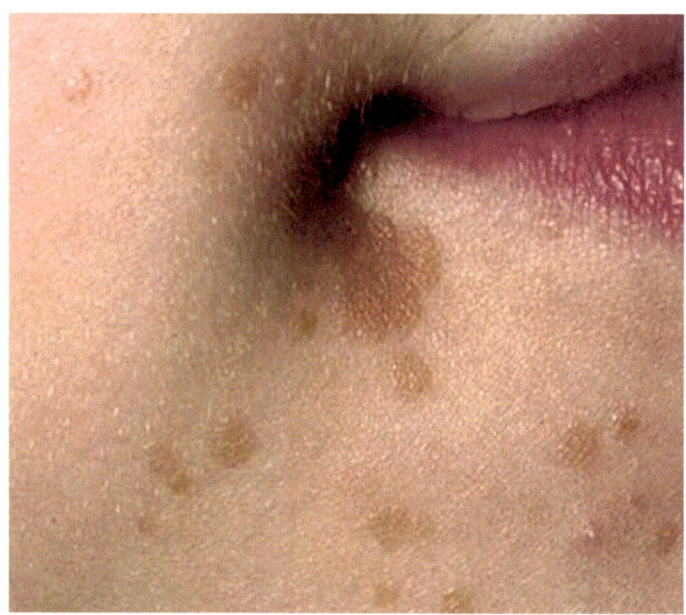

FIGURE 7.1 Verruca plana

Clinical Differential Diagnosis

- Lentigo
- Verruca plana
- Congenital nevus
- Epidermal nevus

Histopathology

A shave biopsy showed slight acanthosis with koilocytic (perinuclear halo clearing) changes in the upper epidermis. The nucleus showed raisinoid (wrinkled) changes (Fig. 7.2).

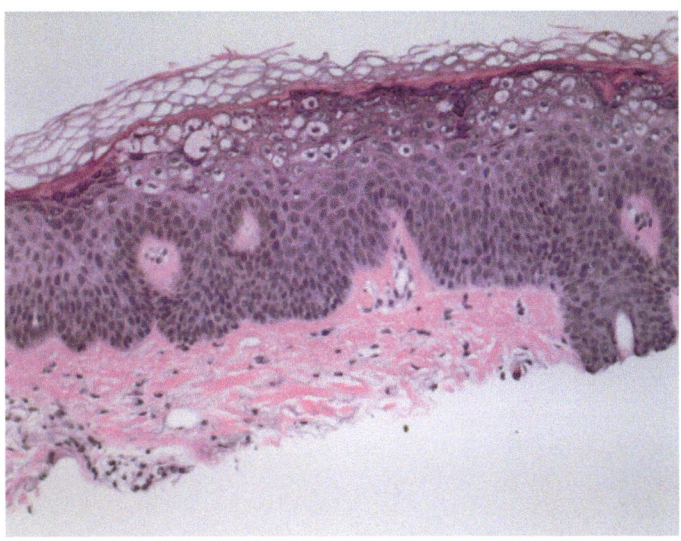

FIGURE 7.2 H&E 100×, Verruca plana shows numerous koilocytes (cytoplasmic clearing), a characteristic feature of HPV infection

Diagnosis

VERRUCA PLANA. It is often referred to as a flat wart and caused by HPV types 3, 10, 28, and 49. Auto-inoculation is a common mode of dissemination.

The flat, tan appearance brings up the differential of a pigmented lesion. Lentigo is due to hyperpigmentation of the basal keratinocytic layer due to increased number of melanocytes. Also a congenital nevus would show larger junction and dermal nests. An epidermal nevus is a type of congenital malformation that shows rudimentary adnexal structures in the dermis.

Treatment Options

- Tacrolimus 0.03 % topical ointment.
- Cantharidin
- Curettage
- Cryotherapy

Recommended Reading

Goldsmith LA et al. Fitzpatrick's dermatology in general medicine. 8th ed. New York: McGraw-Hill Co; 2012. p. 2421–32.

Case 8
25 Year Old White Male with Brown Papillary Growths on Penis

William Eng and Martin J. Walsh

History and Clinical

A 25-year-old-white male presented with multiple growths located on his penile shaft. The patient had a history of genital warts for 4 years that was treated with cryotherapy.

Physical Examination

The patient revealed a brown polypoid growth on the penile shaft (Fig. 8.1).

Clinical Differential Diagnosis

- Epidermal nevus
- Seborrheic keratosis

W. Eng, MD (✉)
Department of Pathology,
University of Central Florida Medical School,
Orlando, FL, USA
e-mail: drwilliameng@yahoo.com

M.J. Walsh, MS, BA
Graduate Studies,
USF College of Medicine, Tampa, FL, USA

R.A. Norman, W. Eng (eds.), *Clinical Cases in Infections and Infestations of the Skin*, Clinical Cases in Dermatology 6, DOI 10.1007/978-3-319-14295-1_8,
© Springer International Publishing Switzerland 2015

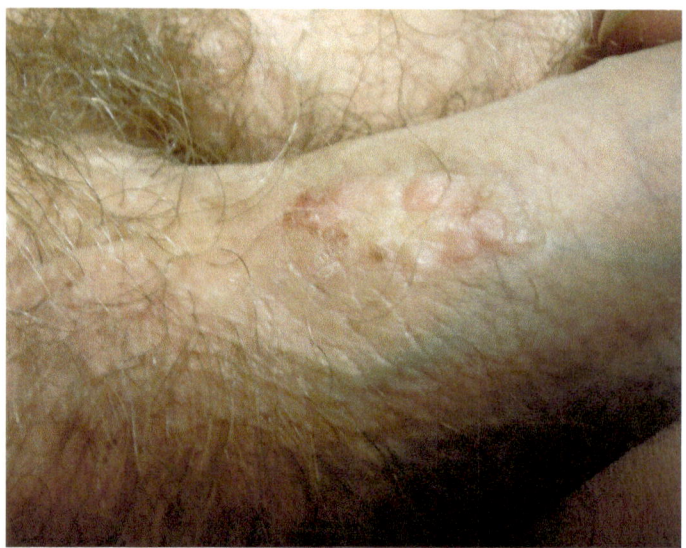

FIGURE 8.1 Condyloma acuminata on patient's penile shaft

- Condyloma acuminata
- Condyloma lata

Histopathology

A shave biopsy was performed on the patient's penile shaft. It measured $0.5 \times 0.3 \times 0.2$ cm. Microscopic sections showed hyperplasia (thickened epithelium) and low papillomatosis that correlated to the cauliflower clinical appearance (Fig. 8.2). Some of the cells showed perinuclear cytoplasmic clearing (koilocytes) with an irregular nuclear contour (Fig. 8.3).

Diagnosis

CONDYLOMA ACUMINATA. This is commonly a sexually transmitted disease that is caused by the Human papilloma virus types 6 and 11.

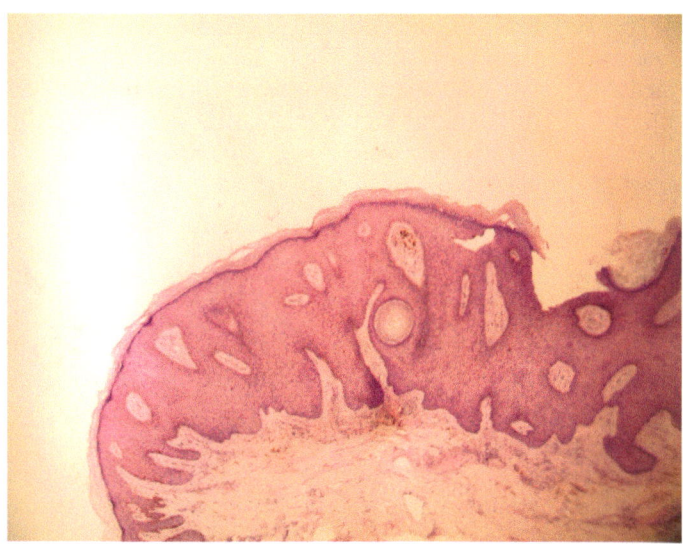

FIGURE 8.2 H&E 40× Condyloma accuminata, acanthosis with low papillomatosis and acanthosis

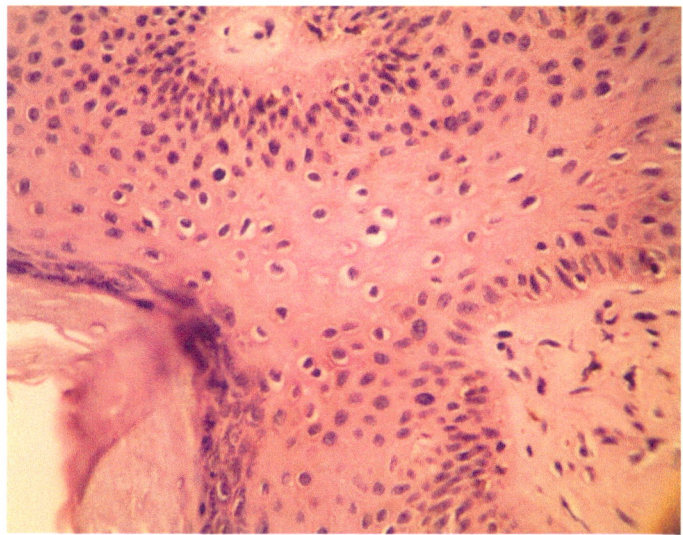

FIGURE 8.3 H&E 400×; Koilocytic changes are characteristic; raisinoid nuclei with cytoplasmic clearing

Epidermal nevus and Seborrheic keratosis both resemble condylomas and each other. While Seborrheic keratosis are acquired, epidermal nevus are congenital in nature. Both lack the koilocytic features, and are negative when probed for HPV virus. Condyloma lata shows epidermal hyperplasia as part of secondary syphilis.

Treatment Options

Although the patient had received cryotherapy on the recurrent genital warts, recurrence is common. The shave biopsy also revealed a fungal infection by *Tinea versicolor*. The patient was prescribed ketoconazole 2 % topical shampoo, ketoconazole 2 % topical cream for his Tinea infection and Podofilox topical 0.5 % topical solution for his genital warts.

Recommended Reading

Goldsmith LA et al. Fitzpatrick's dermatology in general medicine. 8th ed. New York: McGraw-Hill Co; 2012. p. 2421–32.

Case 9
9 Year Old Black Female with Multiple, Small Round, Firm Papules

William Eng and Martin J. Walsh

History and Clinical

A 9-year-old female presented with a recent growth on her chin, left knee and left posterior upper arm. She also had a history of mild acne on her face and lower abdomen. The patient was not on any medications and had no known history of allergies to medications.

Physical Examination

Examination showed several round hyperkeratotic lesions measuring approximately 5 mm in diameter (Figs. 9.1 and 9.2).

W. Eng, MD (✉)
Department of Pathology,
University of Central Florida Medical School, Orlando, FL, USA
e-mail: drwilliameng@yahoo.com

M.J. Walsh, MS, BA
Graduate Studies, USF College of Medicine, Tampa, FL, USA

R.A. Norman, W. Eng (eds.), *Clinical Cases in Infections and Infestations of the Skin*, Clinical Cases in Dermatology 6, DOI 10.1007/978-3-319-14295-1_9,
© Springer International Publishing Switzerland 2015

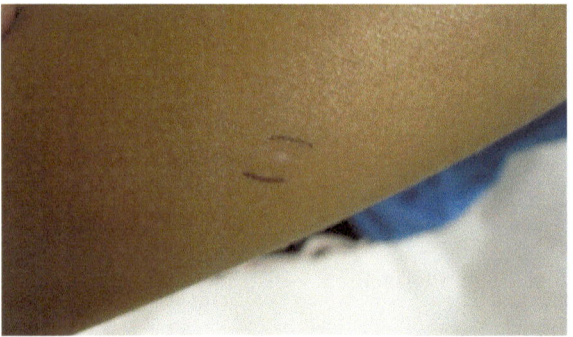

FIGURE 9.1 Verruca vulgaris

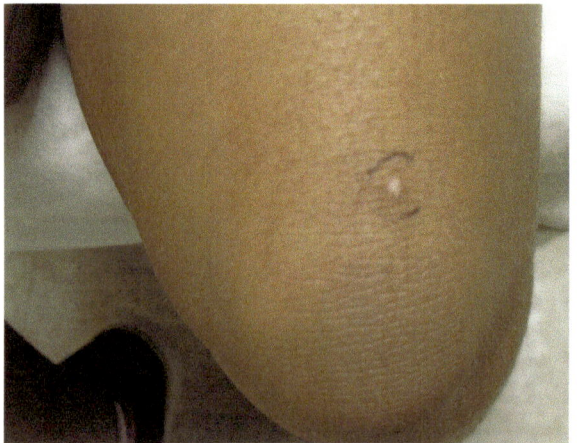

FIGURE 9.2 Verruca vulgaris

Clinical Differential Diagnosis

- Epidermal nevus
- Actinic keratosis
- Seborrheic keratosis
- Verruca vulgaris

Histopathology

The shave biopsy of the left knee was performed and measured $0.3 \times 0.2 \times 0.1$ cm. The left posterior upper arm exhibited slight hyperkeratosis and papillomatosis with acanthosis. Within the epidermis, some keratinocytes exhibited a perinuclear vacuolization with irregular nuclear contours while other keratinocytes exhibited hypergranulotosis. A shave biopsy of the left posterior upper arm was performed and measured $0.3 \times 0.2 \times 0.1$ cm (Figs. 9.1, 9.3, 9.4, and 9.5).

Diagnosis

VERRUCA VULGARIS. This is one of the most common skin lesions encountered in a dermatology clinic, hence its name the "common wart". It is caused by the Human papilloma virus type 2, 4, 27, and 29.

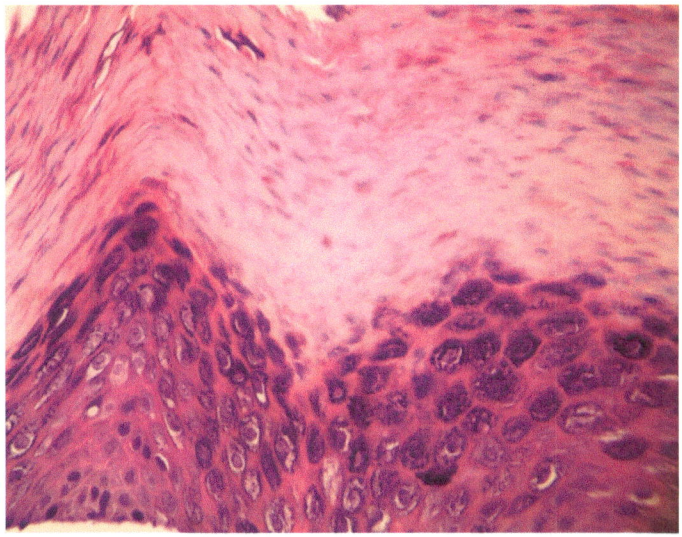

FIGURE 9.3 H&E 400×, Verruca vulgaris, squamous papillomatosis with pointed tip (church spire)

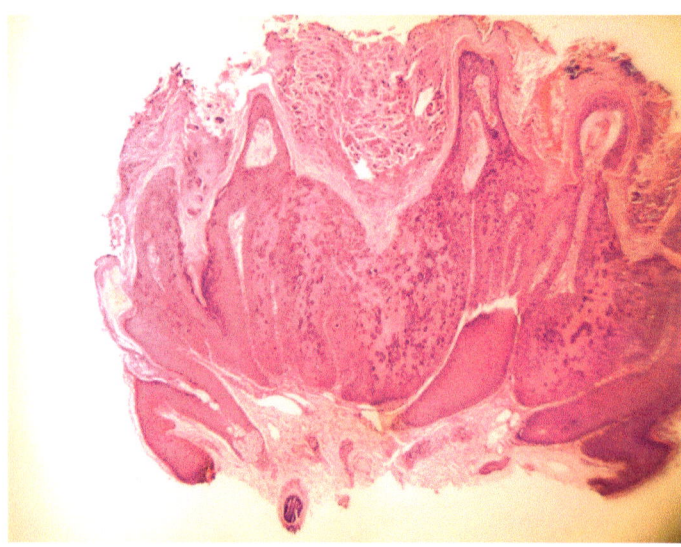

FIGURE 9.4 H&E 40× Verruca vulgaris, prototypical appearance of a wart

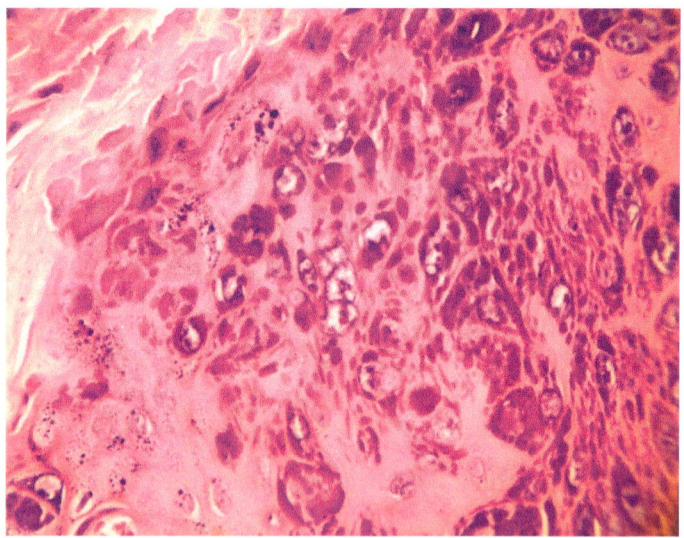

FIGURE 9.5 H&E 400× Verruca vulgaris, Close up of upper epidermis showing hypergranulosis

Seborrheic keratosis and epidermal nevus have both a similar clinical and microscopic appearance. However, verruca features of "church spire" papillomatosis with hypergranulosis are not seen in these two lesions. While actinic keratosis has overlying keratosis like a verruca, it also has basal squamous atypia that is not found in verruca.

Treatment Options

- Cantharidin
- Curettage
- Cryotherapy

Recommended Reading

Goldsmith LA et al. Fitzpatrick's dermatology in general medicine. 8th ed. New York: McGraw-Hill Co; 2012. p. 2421–32.

Case 10
37 Year Old White Male with Multiple, Brown, Purple Nodules on Arms and Legs

William Eng and Martin J. Walsh

History and Clinical

A 37-year-old male presented with lesions on his inferior left arm that had increased in size after starting on HIV medications 2 months prior. The patient also presented with a full body coverage of mildly scaly and pruritic erythematous rash. The patient was positive for HIV and Hepatitis C, but had no known allergies. The patient did mention depressive episodes and weakness. The patient was on the following medications: Amitriptyline HCl 25 mg oral tablet, Hydroxyzine HCl 50 mg oral tablet, Melatonin 1 mg oral tablet, Fluconazole 200 mg oral tablet, Folic Acid 0.8 mg oral tablet, Ritonavir 100 mg oral tablet, Tenofovir/emtricitabine 200 mg-300 mg oral tablet, and Darunavir 800 mg oral tablet.

W. Eng, MD (✉)
Department of Pathology,
University of Central Florida Medical School, Orlando, FL, USA
e-mail: drwilliameng@yahoo.com

M.J. Walsh, MS, BA
Graduate Studies, USF College of Medicine, Tampa, FL, USA

R.A. Norman, W. Eng (eds.), *Clinical Cases in Infections and Infestations of the Skin*, Clinical Cases in Dermatology 6, DOI 10.1007/978-3-319-14295-1_10, © Springer International Publishing Switzerland 2015

Physical Examination

The patient displayed disorientation upon visitation, and he explained that they were side effects of his HIV and hepatitis C medications. He had papular skin eruptions at the inferior portions of his left arm, he showed xerosis at his mid-trunk, and nodules on the superior portions of his left arm, and similar protuberances that covered his legs (Fig. 10.1).

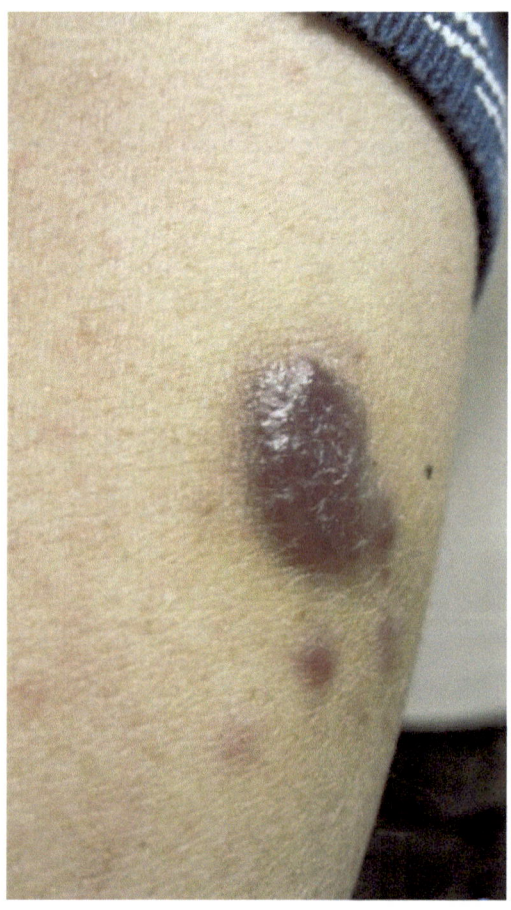

FIGURE 10.1 Kaposi sarcoma presents as a brownish purple nodule

Clinical Differential Diagnosis

- Lymphoma
- Leukemia
- Metastatic malignancy
- Angiosarcoma
- Kaposi sarcoma
- Infection

Histopathology

A 4 mm punch biopsy was performed on the superior left arm. Sections show an ill-defined lesion comprised of short spindled cells. Some of these cells form irregular vascular channels that encircle existing vessels (promotory sign) (Fig. 10.2). While some vessels contain RBCs, other areas show extravasated RBCs with hemosiderin deposits (Fig. 10.3).

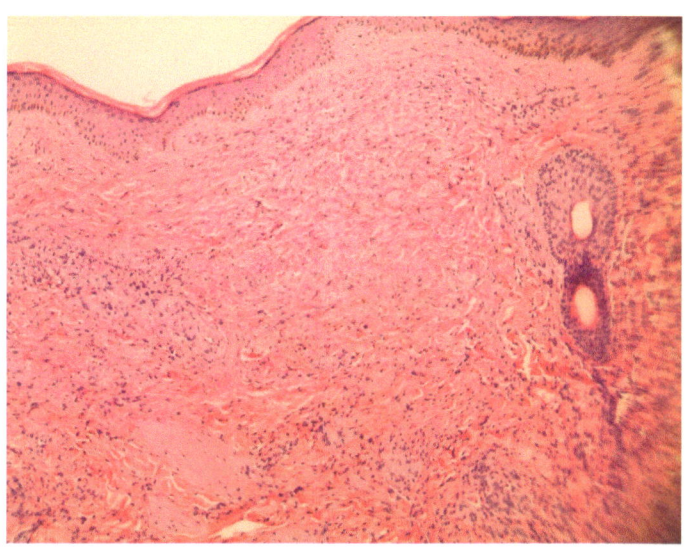

FIGURE 10.2 H&E 100×; Kaposi sarcoma is caused by the HHV8 virus. Multiple slit like vascular channels are found

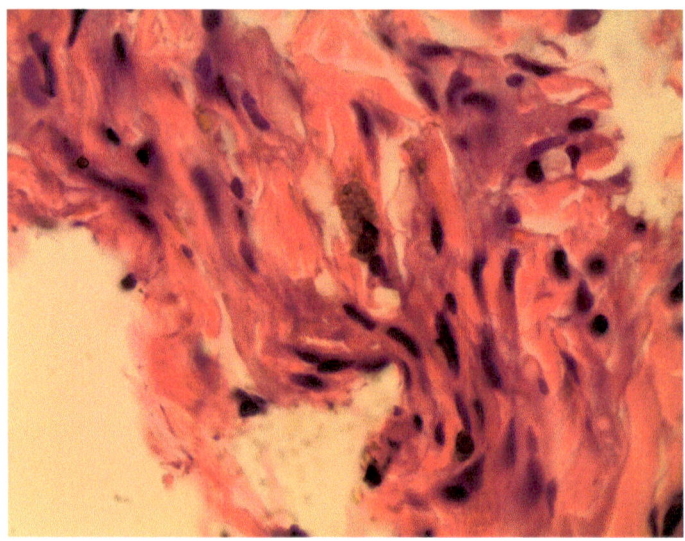

FIGURE 10.3 H&E 1,000×, Kaposi sarcoma, with characteristic hemosiderin deposits

Diagnosis

KAPOSI SARCOMA. In the era before widespread use of HIV antiviral medications, this was a common skin lesion found in AIDS. Today, it is rarely seen unless the patient is noncompliant with his HIV medications. Kaposi sarcoma is not a true malignancy of the soft tissue, but is caused by the HHV8 virus. Another population of non-HIV, elderly patients originating from the Mediterranean or Jewish background have a distinct pattern presentation of Kaposi sarcoma on the lower extremity.

Multiple red-purple nodules brings up the differential of lymphoma and leukemia. Microscopically, both lymphoma and leukemia presents with a near confluence of mononuclear cells. Immunostains can be helpful in classifying the type of lymphoma and leukemia. Metastatic lesions from lung, breast, gastrointestinal, renal, melanoma, and prostate are some of the most common primary sites. Cytokeratin (CK7, CK20), PSA, MART, ER/PR immunostaining is also helpful in this situation as well. Angiosarcoma which is usually solitary on the head and neck region shows markedly atypical cells with areas of immature vascular formation. This tumor is positive for vascular markers (CD31, CD34, Factor 8, vWB) as well as the HHV8 immunostain. Infections microscopically lack the presence of atypical cells, so special stains like PAS, GMS, Gram stains are most helpful along with culture.

Treatment Options

- Chemotherapy; doxorubicin, bleomycin, vincristine, etoposide and dacarbazine
- HAART; Correction of immunodeficiency will often result in regression of Kaposi sarcoma

Recommended Reading

Eng W, Cockerell CJ. Histological features of kaposi sarcoma in a patient receiving highly active antiviral therapy. Am J Dermatopathol. 2004;2:127–32.

Goldsmith LA et al. Fitzpatrick's dermatology in general medicine. 8th ed. New York: McGraw-Hill Co; 2012. p. 1481–86.

Case 11
1 Year Old Male
with Blistering on Mouth
and Palms

William Eng and Lisa M. Diaz

History and Clinical

A 1-year-old male presented with a severe erythematous rash throughout his body. The patient was currently prescribed Mupirocin 2 % topical ointment. There was also a history of eczema eruptions and asthma.

Physical Examination

The patient displayed erythematous papules throughout his body with exorciation and pruritus.

W. Eng, MD (✉)
Department of Pathology,
University of Central Florida Medical School,
Orlando, FL, USA
e-mail: drwilliameng@yahoo.com

L.M. Diaz, DO
Department of Pathology College of Osteopathic Medicine
Lake Erie College of Osteopathic Medicine, Bradenton, FL, USA

R.A. Norman, W. Eng (eds.), *Clinical Cases in Infections and Infestations of the Skin*, Clinical Cases in Dermatology 6, DOI 10.1007/978-3-319-14295-1_11,
© Springer International Publishing Switzerland 2015

Clinical Differential Diagnosis

- Atopic dermatitis
- Allergic contact dermatitis
- Hand Foot Mouth disease

Histopathology

A shave biopsy was performed on the left knee to rule out eczema and scabies. The shave biopsy measured $0.5 \times 0.5 \times 0.1$ cm. The sections of the sample showed marked edematous changes in the epidermis with reticular degeneration. A Periodic-acid Schiff stain tested negative for fungus.

Diagnosis

HAND-FOOT-AND-MOUTH DISEASE (HFMD), otherwise known as vesicular stomatitis with exanthema or coxsackie virus infection, is a highly contagious viral illness that causes an infection characterized by oral stomatitis with a vesicular eruption on the hands and feet. It tends to affect children less than 10 years old but may affect adults also, especially those who are exposed to children within the first week of infection when they are the most contagious. Children less than 5 years old who contract the disease tend to be the most severely affected. The incidence of HFMD increases in the summer and fall months from June to October. In the United States, it is two to three times more likely to occur in the southern states than in the northern states.

The virus is transmitted via respiratory droplets, via the fecal-oral route or via contaminated fomites. Once transmitted, the virus has a 3–6 day incubation period after which symptoms may present. The individual may complain of malaise, sore throat, fever, diarrhea, cough, arthralgia, headaches, and cervical or submandibular lymphadenopathy. Approximately 1–2 days after the initial onset of symptoms the oral lesions appear. These oral lesions characteristically occur on the anterior surface of the tongue, buccal mucosa, gingiva, and hard palate. These lesions evolve from 1 to 3 mm erythematous macules into extremely painful gray vesicles on an erythematous base. Eventually these gray vesicles rupture and form superficial gray ulcers with a surrounding ring of erythema. The typical individual has anywhere from five to ten oral lesions.

The extremities then become involved, with the dorsal hands and dorsal feet being most frequently observed. It is not uncommon for the buttocks and perineum to be involved, as well. The hands are more commonly involved than the feet and these lesions tend to be less painful than those in the mouth. These lesions begin as linear erythematous papules that range in size from 3 to 10 mm in diameter. These papules usually run parallel to skin lines and eventually evolve into gray vesicles that if left alone are resorbed on their own after 2 weeks. Interestingly, only 11 % of adults have cutaneous findings. The disease incidence varies by country and region. In China, HFMD is the most common infectious disease with 91 % of the population affected.

Most cases of HFMD are caused by Coxsackie virus group A type 16. However, HFMD can be caused by any of the following Coxsackie viruses: A5, A7, A9, A10, B1, B2, B3, B5. Enterovirus 71 is also known to cause HFMD and can lead to more severe sequelae. This virus is neurotropic and targets the brainstem resulting in rare and deadly cases of meningitis and encephalitis. It can also cause myocarditis, poliomyelitis-like paralysis, and pulmonary edema. This particular strain is more common in the Asia-Pacific region where it causes many deaths.

The diagnosis of HFMD is usually based on history and physical exam. If a more thorough work up is called for then a throat culture or stool culture can be performed. However, they require 2–4 weeks to obtain results. Reverse Transcriptase Polymerase Chain Reaction can be performed, as well.

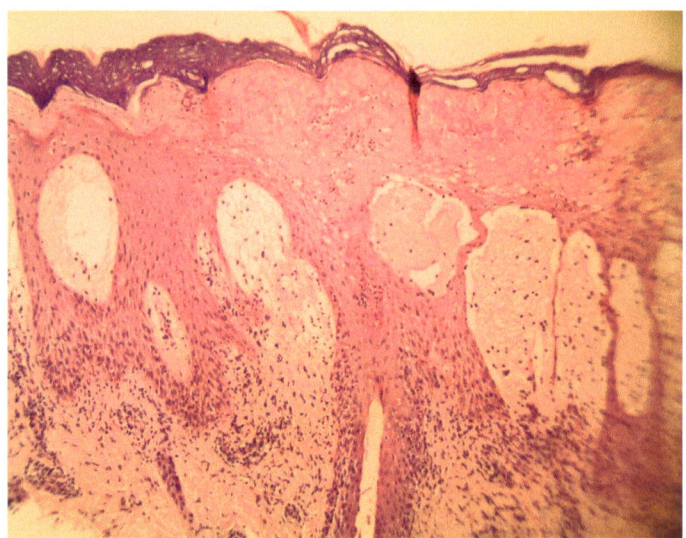

FIGURE 11.1 H&E 400× Hand foot mouth disease

Microscopically, marked intraepidermal vesicles with degeneration changes. The dermis contains a perivascular inflammatory infiltrate with papillary dermal edema (Fig. 11.1). It is more important to rule out any acute serious bacterial infection like meningococcal sepsis that could be causing the manifestation of the lesions.

The changes of allergic or atopic dermatitis which typically contains variable number of eosinophils are not found in this case.

Treatment Options

Hand-foot-and-mouth disease is a self-limiting infection that is typically benign in nature. For this reason, it is treated symptomatically and tends to resolve within 7 days of presentation. Individuals with painful oral lesions may use saltwater rinses, viscous lidocaine mouthwash, and acetaminophen to help control any discomfort. Exposure to the virus does provides immunity but does not prevent future infection by a different viral strain. There are reports of treatment with corticosteroids, intravenous immunoglobulins, and antiviral medications but nothing has been proven to be highly effective thus far. Children diagnosed with a suspected enterovirus 71 infection should be hospitalized immediately and treated accordingly to prevent any central nervous system or cardiac involvement.

Prevention

Due to the highly contagious nature of the disease, frequent hand washing and washing of soiled items is strongly recommended to decrease the spread of this disease. Children with fever, weeping lesions, or those that are actively drooling should be kept from school, day care, or other children. Pregnant women who contract the disease should be seen by an obstetrician who deals with high-risk pregnancies.

Recommended Reading

Ben-Chetrit E, Wiener-Well Y, Shulman LM, et al. Coxsackie A6-related hand foot and mouth disease: skin manifestations in a cluster of adult patients. J Clin Virol. 2014;59(3):201–3.

Ferri FF. "Hand-Foot-Mouth Disease." Ferri's Clinical Advisor. N.p.: Mosby; 2014. p. 474.

Hopper SM, McCarthy M, Tancharoen C, et al. Topical lidocaine to improve oral intake in children with painful infectious mouth ulcers: a blinded, randomized, placebo-controlled trial. Ann Emerg Med. 2014;63:292–9.

Jorizzo JL, Schaffer JV. Dermatology. By Bolognia JL. 3rd ed. N.p.: Elsevier Limited, Waltham, MA; 2012. p. 1345–65.

Kushner D, Caldwell BD. Hand-foot-and-mouth disease. J Am Podiatr Med Assoc. 1996;86(6):257–9.

Lee TC, Guo HR, Su HJ, Yang YC, Chang HL, Chen KT. Diseases caused by enterovirus 71 infection. Pediatr Infect Dis J. 2009;28:904–10.

Ooi MH, Wong SC, Mohan A, et al. Identification and validation of clinical predictors for the risk of neurological involvement in children with hand, foot, and mouth disease in Sarawak. BMC Infect Dis. 2009;9:3.

Prager P, Nolan M, Andrews IP, Williams GD. Neurogenic pulmonary edema in enterovirus 71 encephalitis is not uniformly fatal but causes severe morbidity in survivors. Pediatr Crit Care Med. 2003;4:377–81.

Shi RX, Wang JF, Lai X, et al. Spatiotemporal pattern of hand-foot-mouth disease in China: an analysis of empirical orthogonal functions. Public Health. 2014;128(4):367–75.

Case 12
46 Year Old Male with Necrotic Blisters on Hands

William Eng and Lisa M. Diaz

History and Clinical

A 46 year old hunter presented with a multiple, painful lesions on his hands. He was on a recent deer hunting trip where he butchered several deer that his hunting party had shot.

Physical Examination

Examination showed multiple irregular zones of necrosis on the acral surface of his hands. He was afebrile and alert.

Clinical Differential Diagnosis

- Herpes
- Irritant contact dermatitis
- Orf

W. Eng, MD (✉)
Department of Pathology,
University of Central Florida Medical School, Orlando, FL, USA
e-mail: drwilliameng@yahoo.com

L.M. Diaz, DO
Lake Erie College of Osteopathic Medicine, Bradenton, FL, USA

R.A. Norman, W. Eng (eds.), *Clinical Cases in Infections and Infestations of the Skin*, Clinical Cases in Dermatology 6, DOI 10.1007/978-3-319-14295-1_12, © Springer International Publishing Switzerland 2015

Diagnosis

ORF, or ecthyma contagiosum, is an infection caused by parapoxvirus. When humans are infected, inflammation and necrosis occur at the site of inoculation. Sheep, goats, and deer are the natural reservoirs of the virus. Humans who are bitten by infected animals or who are exposed to contaminated fomites can contract the disease. It tends to affect individuals who work as farmers, butchers, veterinarians, and sheepherders. The most commonly affected sites of direct contact, namely the fingers, hands, arms, and elbows.

After an incubation period of 5 days, an erythematous or blue papule forms at the site of viral entry. The papule evolves into a flat-topped pustule, may be numerous, and can grow up to 4 cm in size. Accompanying symptoms include: mild fever, regional lymphadenopathy, and tenderness.

Orf is a viral infection that proceeds through six distinct stages, each of which lasts approximately 6 days. The stages progress in the following order: maculopapular, target, acute weeping nodular, regenerative, papillomatous, and regressive (Figs. 12.1 and 12.2).

There are reported cases of Orf infection triggering erythema multiforme, secondary bacterial infections, generalized papular or morbilliform reactions, as well as blistering eruptions similar to bullous pemphigoid in affected individuals. Some studies are arguing that these bullous eruptions observed after Orf infections are distinct autoimmune diseases.

The diagnosis is usually made based on history and physical examination. If a more thorough work up is required, electron microscopy may be performed on a scraping of the lesion. Also, a biopsy or polymerase chain reaction for viral RNA can be diagnostic. A herpes infection can identified by finding keratinocytes with multiple nuclei molded together. An irritant contact dermatitis can be elicited from the clinical history and extensive necrosis with neutrophils.

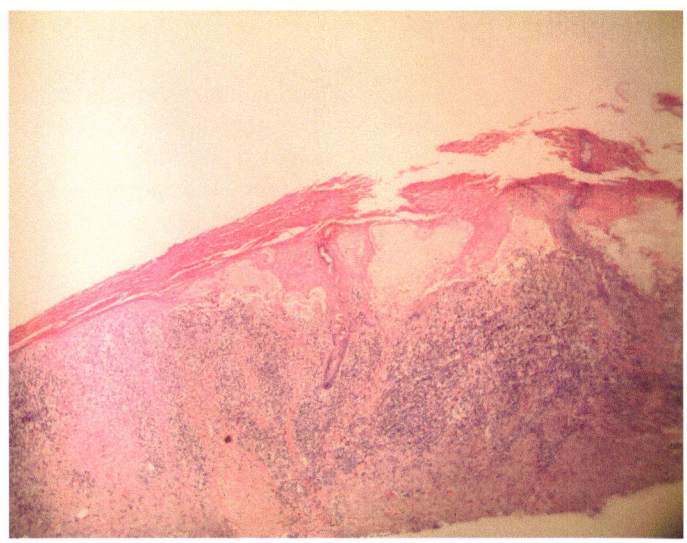

FIGURE 12.1 H&E 40×, ORF

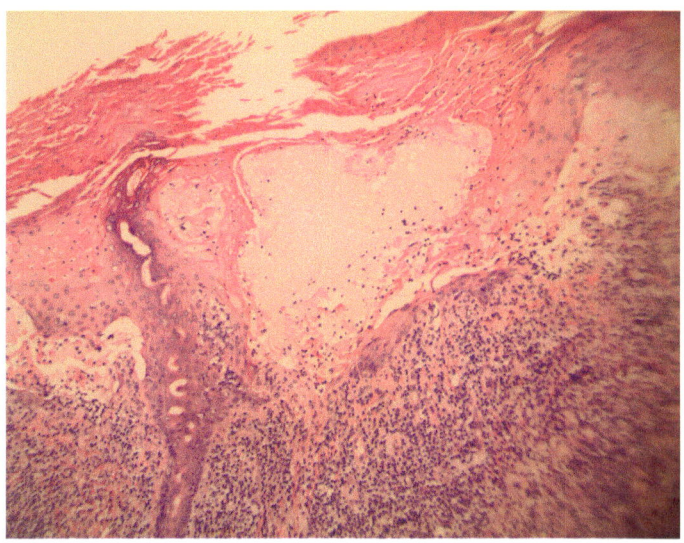

FIGURE 12.2 H&E 100×, ORF

Treatment Options

Orf is typically a self-limiting infection that requires only supportive care. Most cases resolve completely within 2–7 weeks. Treatment only becomes necessary if secondary bacterial infection occurs or if the patient is immunocompromised.

Surgery and cryotherapy may be used to help debulk the infected tissue. There are also reports of using idoxuridine and cidofovir for either shortening healing time or help clear persistent infections. Other more recent therapies that could be considered include imiquimod cream and interferon.

Prevention

Preventative measures are key in disease management. Sheep may be vaccinated to help boost their immune response and reduce the viral reservoir. Also, those who work with sheep are strongly recommended to wear gloves and protective clothing when there is any suspicion that the animal may be infected.

Recommended Reading

Candiani JO, Soto RG, Lozano OW. Orf nodule: treatment with cryosurgery. J Am Acad Dermatol. 1993;29:256–7.

Hawkins CN, Tremaine R. An unusual case of orf on the face. J Am Acad. 2013;68(4):AB132.

Lebwohl MG, Heymann WR, John B, Ian C. "Orf." Treatment of skin disease: comprehensive therapeutic strategies. 4th ed. N.p.: Waltham: Elsevier Limited; 2014. p. 519–20.

Leavell UW, McNamara MJ, Muelling R, et al. Orf. Report of 19 human cases with clinical and pathological observations. JAMA. 1968;204:657–64.

Tan ST, Blake GB, Chambers S. Recurrent orf in an immunocompromised host. Br J Plast Surg. 1991;44:465–7.

Torfason EG, Gudnadottir SJ. Polymerase chain reaction for laboratory diagnosis of orf virus infections. Clin Virol. 2002;24:79–84.

White KP, Zedek DC, White WL, et al. Orf-induced immunobullous disease: a distinct autoimmune blistering disorder. J Am Acad Dermatol. 2008;58(1):49–55.

Part II
Bacterial

Case 13
18 Year Old Female with Crusty, Perioral Lesion

William Eng and Lisa M. Diaz

History and Clinical

A 18 year old female presented with a weeping, crusty lesion for the past few days around the right corner of her mouth.

Physical Examination

A yellowish crusted material was seen over an erythematous base (Fig. 13.1). At the periphery, a viscous white-yellowish fluid was found oozing. The area was tender to touch, but not very painful. The patient was also in the first trimester of her pregnancy.

W. Eng, MD (✉)
Department of Pathology,
University of Central Florida Medical School, Orlando, FL, USA
e-mail: drwilliameng@yahoo.com

L.M. Diaz, DO
Lake Erie College of Osteopathic Medicine, Bradenton, FL, USA

R.A. Norman, W. Eng (eds.), *Clinical Cases in Infections
and Infestations of the Skin*, Clinical Cases in Dermatology 6,
DOI 10.1007/978-3-319-14295-1_13,
© Springer International Publishing Switzerland 2015

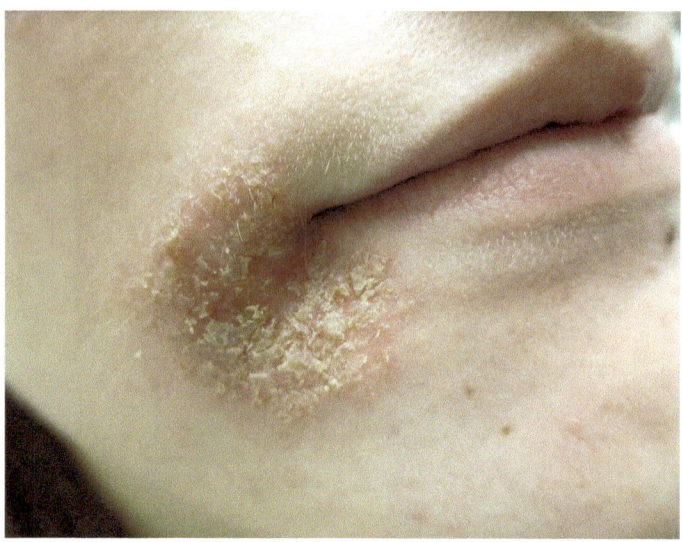

FIGURE 13.1 Impetigo, a "honey crusted" covering an erythematous base

Clinical Differential Diagnosis

- Impetigo
- Contact dermatitis
- Scabies
- Candidiasis

Diagnosis

IMPETIGO (bacterial) is a common infection of the skin that is highly contagious. It is divided into two categories: nonbullous and bullous impetigo. Nonbullous impetigo is the more common form that is responsible for 70 % of cases and occurs in individuals of all ages. It is usually caused by *Staphylococcus aureus* or Group A beta-hemolytic *streptococcus* (*Streptococcus pyogenes*). The lesions begin as vesicles

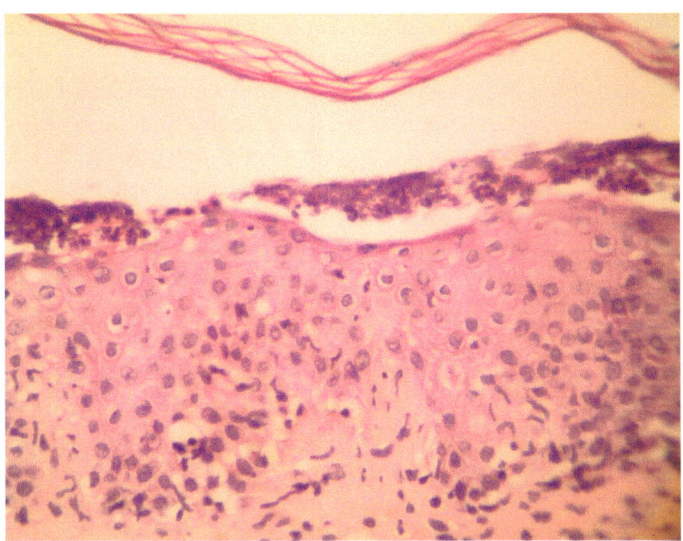

FIGURE 13.2 H&E 100×. Bacteria infection, Impetigo

that quickly rupture and produce a characteristic honey-colored crust.

Bullous impetigo is caused by *Staphylococcus aureus* and is more likely to affect neonates and older infants. These lesions also begin as vesicles that quickly enlarge to form bullae containing clear or yellowish fluid. After 2 or 3 days these bullae rupture and form light brown crusts that border erythematous erosions. The lesions are usually painless and heal without scarring. Some patients complain of pruritus or a burning sensation. Microscopically, the vesicle is separated at the level of the stratum corneum which contains a few trapped neutrophils (Fig. 13.2).

Impetigo usually occurs around the nose and the mouth and is also frequently seen on exposed extremities. It develops at sites of minor skin trauma like abrasions that permit "impetiginzation" or introduction of the infection. Impetigo tends to affect individuals with compromised skin barriers and immune systems like those with atopic dermatitis and diabetes. Streptococcal impetigo is seen more often in warm, humid climates, during the summer months, and spreads quickly in overcrowded environments.

In bullous impetigo, *S aureus* produces an exfoliative toxin that causes the development of the bulla. Methicillin-resistant *S aureus* is becoming an increasingly common etiologic agent. In industrialized countries, mixed infections are becoming more frequent, as well. Typically the infection begins as a streptococcal infection that is then secondarily infected by *S aureus*.

Impetigo is a clinical diagnosis. A work up is unnecessary unless MRSA is suspected and then a culture can be performed with antibiotic sensitivities and resistance. A contact dermatitis could have a similar clinical and microscopic appearance, but microscopically there would be no bacteria seen by special stains.

Treatment

For most cases of impetigo, topical mupirocin treatment is usually sufficient. In cases of infections over a large surface area, fever, complicating cellulitis or other systemic systems, oral therapy can be started. Topical mupirocin is a safe option with published success rates of greater than 90 %. It is applied topically to the affected area three times a day. In order for the topical treatment to be effective, the affected area must be washed with antibacterial soap and wiped with wet compresses to remove the crust. All orifices in the vicinity of the infection, particularly the nares are often reservoirs of bacteria. So these areas should be treated with mupirocin to prevent recurrent infection. A novel formulation that consistent of plant extracts has been shown to exhibit potent anti-microbial activity against a broad spectrum of Gram positive and negative organisms, including MRSA.

Retapamulin is a newer topical antibiotic on the market. It is approved for the treatment of impetigo caused by *S aureus* or *S pyogenes* in adults and children older than 9 months. A large meta-analysis found it to be as effective or slightly more effective than systemic therapy with erythromycin. Non-MRSA oral antibiotics include erythromycin, cephalexin, and amoxicillin-clavulanate. In cases of MRSA infection, coverage can be provided with TMP-SMX, doxycycline, clindamycin or linezolid.

Prevention

Due to its highly contagious nature, good personal hygiene is strongly recommended. Close contacts and household members are at increased risk of acquiring infection. Also at risk are individuals who are team members and share sports equipment. It is recommended that children with impetigo stay home for the first 24 h after beginning antibiotic treatment to reduce the risk of spread to other children. Scratching should be discouraged to decrease the likelihood of auto-inoculation.

Recommended Reading

Bolaji RS, Dabade TS, Gustafson CJ, et al. Treatment of impetigo: oral antibiotics most commonly prescribed. J Drugs Dermatol. 2012;11:489–94.

Eng W, Norman R. Development of an oregano-based ointment with anti-microbial activity including activity against methicillin-resistant Staphylococcus aureus. J Drugs Dermatol. 2010;9(4): 377–80.

George A, Rubin G. A systematic review and meta-analysis of treatments for impetigo. Br J Gen Pract. 2003;53:480–7.

Habif TP. Skin disease (Campbell JL, Chapman MS, Dinulos JGH, Zug KA, editors). 3rd ed. N.p.: Waltham: Elsevier; 2011. p. 154–83.

Lebwohl MF, Heymann WR, John B, Ian C. Treatment of skin disease: comprehensive therapeutic strategies. 4th ed. N.p.: Waltham: Elsevier; 2014. p. 332–4.

Koning S, van der Wouden JC, Chosidow O, et al. Efficacy and safety of retapamulin ointment as treatment of impetigo: randomized double-blind multicentre placebo-controlled trial. Br J Dermatol. 2008;158:1077–82.

Laupland KB, Conly JM. Treatment of Staphylococcus aureus colonization and prophylaxis for infection with topical intranasal mupirocin: an evidence-based review. Clin Infect Dis. 2003;37: 933–8.

Mertz PM, Marshall DA, Eaglstein WH, et al. Topical mupirocin treatment of impetigo is equal to oral erythromycin therapy. Arch Dermatol. 1989;125:1069–73.

Yang LP, Keam SJ. Retapamulin: a review of its use in the management of impetigo and other uncomplicated superficial skin infections. Drugs. 2008;68(6):855–73.

Case 14
70 Year Old Asian Male with Multiple, Erythematous Lesions that Have Decreased Sensation

William Eng and Lisa M. Diaz

History and Clinical

A 70 year old Asian male presented with multiple rashes. He had recently traveled to the India countryside.

Physical Examination

The patient presented with multiple round to oval shaped rashes with loss of pin-prick sensation in the center.

W. Eng, MD (✉)
Department of Pathology,
University of Central Florida Medical School, Orlando, FL, USA
e-mail: drwilliameng@yahoo.com

L.M. Diaz, DO
Lake Erie College of Osteopathic Medicine, Bradenton, FL, USA

R.A. Norman, W. Eng (eds.), *Clinical Cases in Infections and Infestations of the Skin*, Clinical Cases in Dermatology 6, DOI 10.1007/978-3-319-14295-1_14,
© Springer International Publishing Switzerland 2015

Clinical Differential Diagnosis

(Annular rash pattern)

- Mycosis fungoides
- Subacute lupus
- Tinea (ringworm)
- Hansen's disease (Leprosy)
- Syphilis

Diagnosis

HANSEN'S DISEASE, commonly known as leprosy, is a disease caused by Mycobacterium leprae, a slow-growing, acid-fast bacillus with an affinity for cooler regions of the body. These regions include peripheral nerves, skin in non-intertriginous area, testes, and the anterior chambers of the eye. The clinical presentation of leprosy varies depending on the disease state. In 1966, Ridley and Jopling divided the disease activity spectrum of leprosy into distinct forms that are still used today. These forms take into account the host's immunopathologic response to M. leprae and are listed in order by decreasing cell-mediated immunity and increasing disease severity: Tuberculoid leprosy (TT), Borderline tuberculoid leprosy (BT), Midborderline leprosy (BB), Borderline lepromatous leprosy (BL) and Lepromatous leprosy (LL) (Fig. 14.1).

Tuberculoid leprosy represents the immunologically stable, pauci-bacillary form of the disease. It is characterized by a strong cellular response with a weak humoral response from the host. There is typically one large, anesthetic erythematous macule or hypopigmented plaque with a well-defined border and atrophic center that may be found on the face or limbs but usually not on the scalp or in the intertriginous regions. The lesions seen in BT are more abundant and smaller in size with peripheral spread and resolving centers. Thickened nerves and loss of function are commonly seen especially with the greater auricular

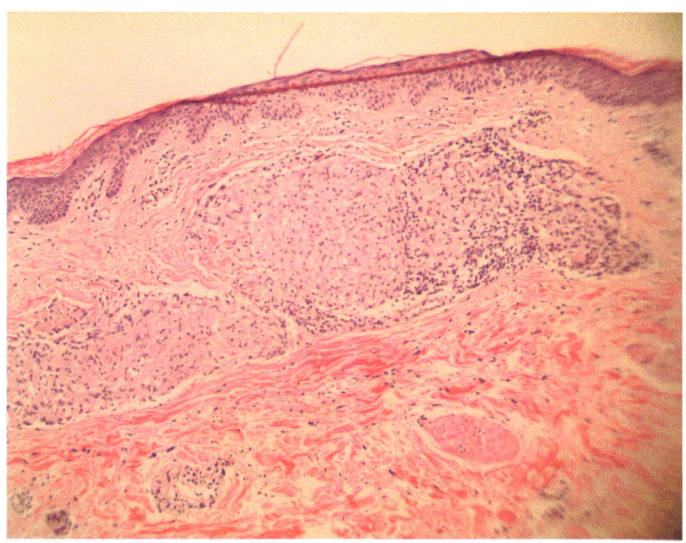

FIGURE 14.1 H&E 100× Leprosy. A granulomatous inflammation with scant lymphocytic infiltrates (Polar Tuberculoid Leprosy pattern)

and superficial peroneal nerves. Patients with mid border-line leprosy present with sharply defined annular plaques. Patients with BL have a varied presentation with multiple, symmetrical macules, papules, and nodules found anywhere on the body. These lesions sometimes appear "punched out" and are hypesthetic. The TT is considered the stable form and appear as sharply defined, reddish-brown plaques. The LL form represents systemic involvement, but in the skin, symmetrical, multiple small macules, plaques with poorly defined borders.

Leprosy causes peripheral neuropathy that affects small nerve fibers that convey temperature, touch, pain, and deep pressure. Lepra reactions occur when there is an acute change in the patient's immune status. The lepra reactions are divided into Type 1 and Type 2. Type 1 lepra reactions consist of swelling of previous plaques and sudden development of new nodules. This type of reaction can be seen in any form of leprosy but is most common in the borderline leprosy stage. Type 2 lepra reactions are also referred to as erythema nodosum leprosum (ENL) and are characterized by tender pink nodules on the extremities with systemic symptoms that may include fever, arthralgias, neuritic pain, uveitis, and orchitis. This reaction only occurs in BL and LL patients.

Pathology

The majority of cases are found in Brazil, Nepal, India, Burma, Indonesia, and Madagascar. The cases reported in the United States are typically due to vacationers traveling in endemic regions or immigrants moving from those countries. It is transmitted by respiratory droplets and requires close contact for an extended period of time in order to acquire the disease. The incubation period of M. leprae spans 5–30 years. Armadillos, chimpanzees, and managabey monkeys are animal reservoirs for the bacillus.

The diagnosis of leprosy can be confirmed using slit skin smears, skin biopsy with acid-fast stains, polymerase chain reaction or peripheral nerve biopsy. Mycosis fungoides has an annular appearance, but microscopically there is a proliferation of atypical lymphocytes found in the epidermis that shows minimal spongiosis. These lymphocytes can either be CD4 or CD8 positive. T cell gene rearrangement studies can be done for confirmation. Another annular lesion is subacute lupus. Lupus presents microscopically with an interface lymphocytic infiltrates with some dermal mucin. Direct immunofluorescent studies may show granular deposits of IgG, IgM and fibrin. Serological studies for ANA can be performed. Tinea corporis is readily diagnosed by a PAS or GMS staining which reveals multiple fungal elements within the cornified layer whereas syphilis typically has numerous plasma cells.

Treatment Options

Leprosy is curable with a multi-drug treatment regimen of dapsone, rifampin, and clofazimine for a period of 6–12 months. Once the patient is being treated they are no longer contagious. Patients experiencing lepra reactions can be treated with corticosteroids.

Prevention

Avoid travel to endemic areas or close contact with infected individuals. Those diagnosed with lepromatous leprosy are the most contagious and household family members should be treated simultaneously.

Recommended Reading

1. Bolognia JL. Mycobacterial Infections. In: Jorizzo JL, Schaffer JV, editors. Dermatology. 3rd ed. N.p.: Waltham: Elsevier; 2012. p. 1221–42.
2. Ferri FF, Johnson L, Opal SM, Harper W, Mylonakis EE. "Leprosy." Ferri's Clinical Advisor. N.p.: St Louis: Mosby; 2014.
3. James WD, Berger TG, Elston DM. Hansen's disease. In: James WD, editor. Andrews' diseases of the skin clinical dermatology. 11th ed. N.p.: Waltham: Elsevier; 2011. p. 334–44.

Case 15
46 Year Old Female with Multiple Slightly Eroded Reddish Papules on Her Arm

William Eng and Martin J. Walsh

History and Clinical

A 46-year-old female presented with a growth on the superior right arm that had been present for 9 months. The patient had a history of a cholecystectomy and tubal ligation. A lipoma was noted on a past physical exam, but it was not removed. She was in prison 5 years ago where she contracted tuberculosis, but failed to complete the course of antibiotics prescribed.

Physical Examination

Examination of the patient exhibited a prominent lipoma at her medial hypogastric region. The patient also presented with an ichthyotic lesion on her right forearm and acrochordons at her bilateral superior axilla and medial hypogastric regions. The right arm showed multiple, red papules, some of which were eroded.

W. Eng, MD (✉)
Department of Pathology,
University of Central Florida Medical School, Orlando, FL, USA
e-mail: drwilliameng@yahoo.com

M.J. Walsh, MS, BA
Graduate Studies, USF College of Medicine, Tampa, FL, USA

R.A. Norman, W. Eng (eds.), *Clinical Cases in Infections and Infestations of the Skin*, Clinical Cases in Dermatology 6, DOI 10.1007/978-3-319-14295-1_15, © Springer International Publishing Switzerland 2015

Clinical Differential Diagnosis

- Syphilis
- Sporotrichosis
- Tularemia
- Bartonellosis
- Mycobacterium
- Tuberulosis

Histopathology

A shave biopsy was performed on the patient's superior right arm (Fig. 15.1). The biopsy measured $0.6 \times 0.6 \times 0.5$, and a separate piece measured $0.7 \times 0.6 \times 0.1$ cm. This specimen tested negative for fungus in by Periodic Acid-Schiff stain. The microscopic presentation showed a central oval area of necrosis that was surrounded by a prominent histocytes and multi-nucleated giant cells (Figs. 15.2, 15.3, and 15.4). The Acid Fast Stain showed numerous positive staining organisms with a short rod appearance (Fig. 15.5).

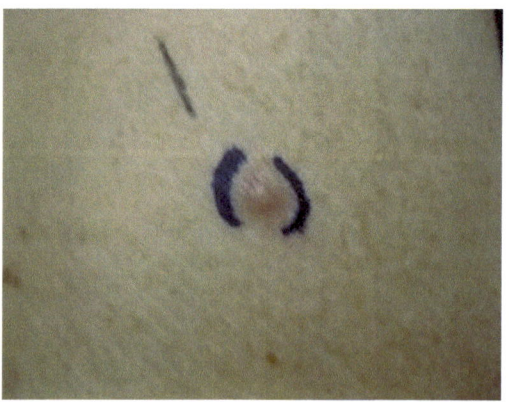

FIGURE 15.1 Mycobacterium tuberculosis

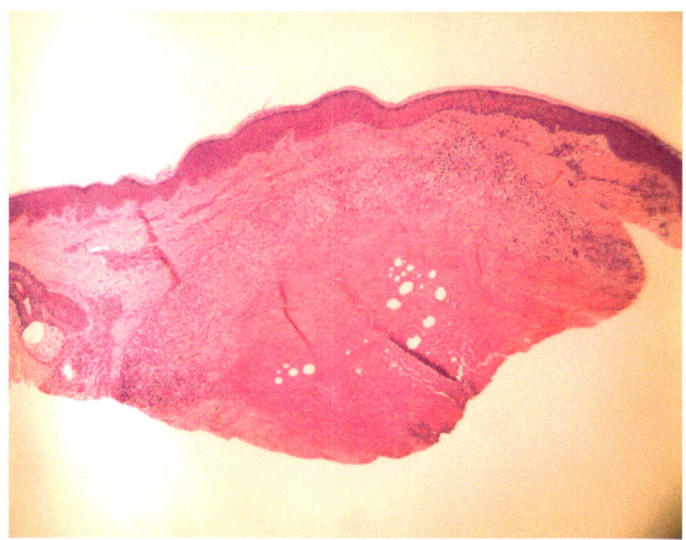

FIGURE 15.2 H&E 40× discrete subcutaneous nodule

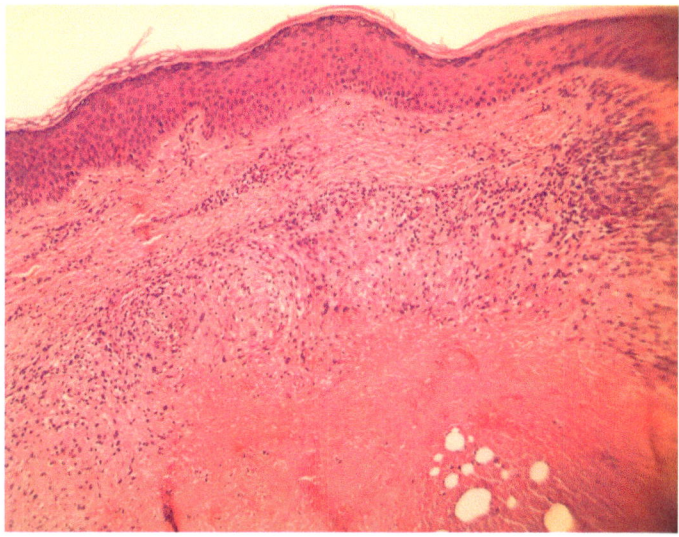

FIGURE 15.3 H&E 100×, Outer wall consists of lymphocytes and histiocytes while the center is necrotic

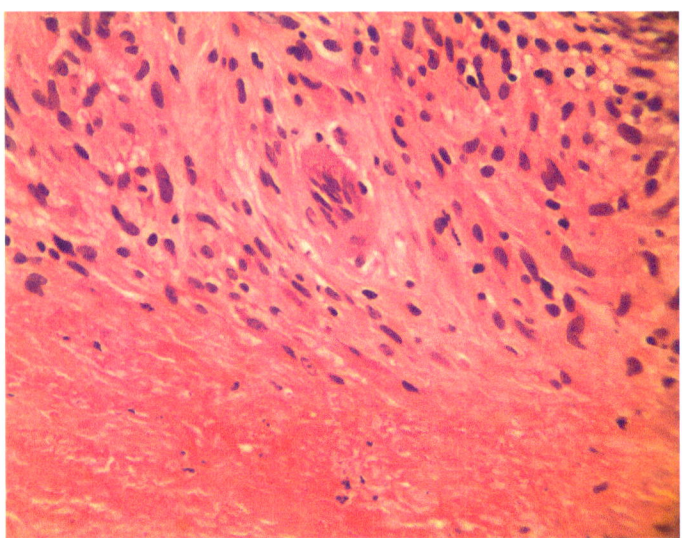

FIGURE 15.4 H&E 400×, Scattered multinucleate giants cells are found within outer wall

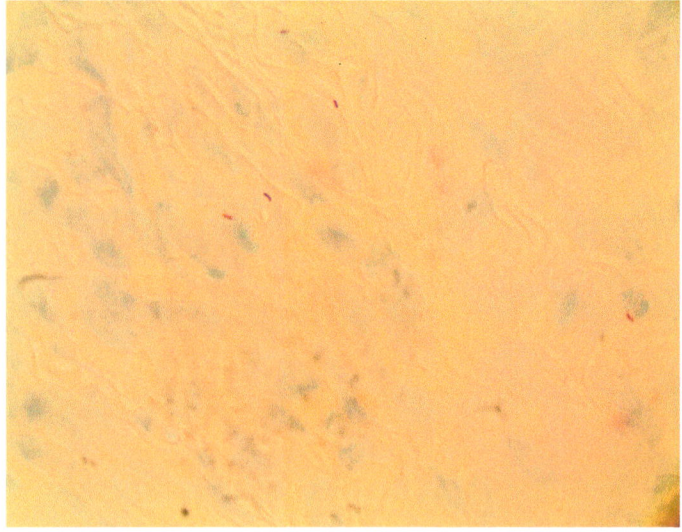

FIGURE 15.5 Acid fast bacilli stain, 1,000× scattered small, rod-shaped bacteria (*red*) are found within the central necrosis

Diagnosis

MYCOBACTERIUM TUBERCULOSIS. Tuberculosis remains a world-wide disease with a third of the world population being infected. Most new infections are arising from Africa. HIV positive patients are at a 20× increased risk of contracting tuberculosis. The organism can be disseminated into all organs, but in the skin it often appears as "lupus vulgaris" or "scrofuloderma". The organism grows intracellularly, and induces a granulomatous reaction.

While infectious processes can have a similar clinical appearance, microscopic examination using special stains as well as immunostains aid in the identification of a specific organisms. Although tissue cultures remain the traditional method of separating certain species based on metabolic features, newer molecular techniques are gaining acceptance. Clinically, the "B" symptoms are associated with tuberculosis; weight loss, night sweats, and fever. A chest x-ray is helpful in evaluating for pulmonary disease.

Treatment Options

Treatment is usually a combination therapy

- Isoniazide
- Rifamycin
- Pyrazinamide
- Ethambutol

Recommended Reading

Goldsmith LA. Fitzpatrick's dermatology in general medicine. 8th ed. New York: McGraw-Hill Co; 2012. p. 2225–40.

Case 16
56 Year Old Black Male with Multiple Draining Pustules and Nodules on Posterior Neck and Scalp

William Eng and Lisa M. Diaz

History and Clinical

A 56 year black male presented with a rash on the back of his neck. The lesion began shortly after visiting his barber who had given him a customized, short haircut.

Physical Examination

The patient showed multiple papules and nodules, some of which were expressing pus. The affected area also had a firm boggy consistency that was extremely tender to the touch (Fig. 16.1).

W. Eng, MD (✉)
Department of Pathology,
University of Central Florida Medical School, Orlando, FL, USA
e-mail: drwilliameng@yahoo.com

L.M. Diaz, DO
Lake Erie College of Osteopathic Medicine, Bradenton, FL, USA

R.A. Norman, W. Eng (eds.), *Clinical Cases in Infections and Infestations of the Skin*, Clinical Cases in Dermatology 6, DOI 10.1007/978-3-319-14295-1_16,
© Springer International Publishing Switzerland 2015

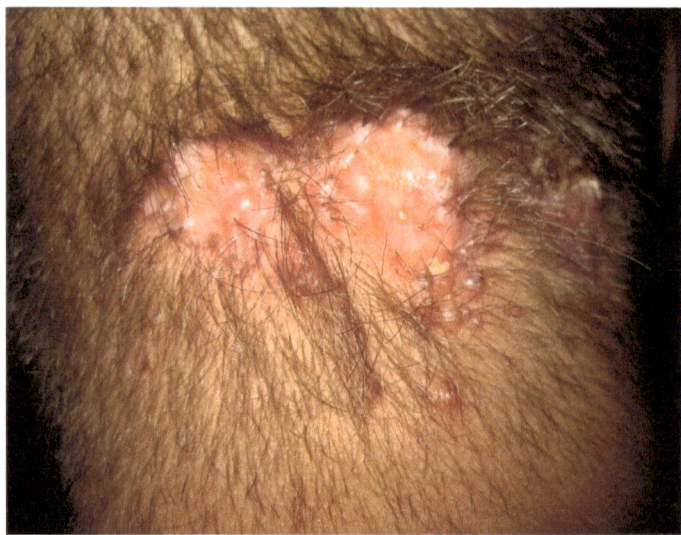

FIGURE 16.1 Posterior neck showing folliculitis (Sycosis nuchae)

Clinical Differential Diagnosis

- Folliculitis
- Adnexal tumor
- Cysts
- Acne keloidalis

Diagnosis

FOLLICULITIS is defined as inflammation of the pilosebaceous unit (Fig. 16.2). Clinically, it appears as folliculocentric papules or pustules on an erythematous base. Folliculitis can be asymptomatic but the patient may complain of tenderness, pain or pruritus. If the pruritus becomes generalized it is referred to as "itching folliculitis." Typically the lesions are distributed in areas where terminal hairs are found such as the scalp, beard, upper trunk, buttocks and lower extremities.

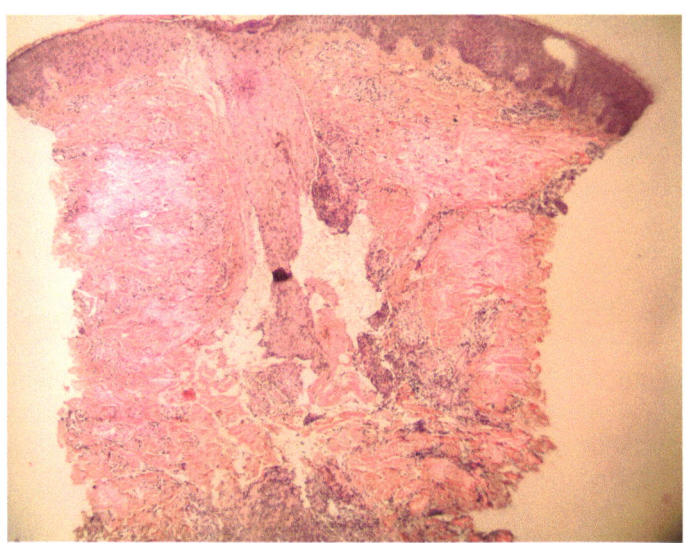

FIGURE 16.2 H&E 40×, Central hair follicle is surrounded by mixed inflammation

The bacterial etiology of folliculitis can be divided into two groups, those caused by gram-positive bacteria and those caused by gram-negative bacteria. The majority of cases of bacterial folliculitis are caused by *Staphylococcus aureus*. In the past, *methicillin-resistant Staphylococcus aureus* (MRSA) was more likely to be present in the form of cellulitis. However, the incidence of MRSA folliculitis is on the rise. Fortunately, MRSA cellullitis and *methicillin-sensitive Staphylococcus aureus* (MSSA) folliculitis have clinically distinct presentations and this helps dermatologists in making the accurate diagnosis. MSSA folliculitis is still more common and tends to be found in the axillary region, beard, buttocks, and extremities of patients. In contrast, MRSA folliculitis appears in a more atypical distribution around the umbilicus, chest, flank, and scrotum.

Folliculitis caused by *Staphylococcus* is more likely to occur in patients who are immunocompromised, hyperhidrotic, atopic or who have a history of **MRSA** infections. Those individuals are likely to be chronic nasal *Staphylococcus* carriers and prone to recurrent infections. When *Staphylococcus* infects the hair follicles in the beard region, it is referred to as sycosis barbae. If it affects the posterior neck, it is called sycosis nuchae.

Gram-negative rods make up the second group of bacteria that can cause folliculitis. This collection of bacteria includes the *Klebsiella*, *Escherichia coli*, *Proteus*, and *Enterobacter* species. Follicular infection by gram-negative bacteria is less common than infection from *S. aureus*. However, cases of gram-negative bacteria tend to be more recalcitrant and difficult to eradicate. Most cases of gram-negative folliculitis are secondary to long-term use of oral tetracyclines for acne treatment.

Another gram-negative microbe that causes folliculitis is *Pseudomonas aeruginosa*. Also referred to as "hot tub folliculitis" *P. aeruginosa* is responsible for the acute onset of folliculitis 12–48 h after the use of a contaminated hot tub. These lesions tend to be more edematous in appearance. A study published by Lutz and Lee demonstrated the recent increase in multi-drug resistant *P. aeruginosa*. The study showed that 96 % of the *P. aeruginosa* organisms taken from swimming pools and hot tubs exhibited multi-drug resistance.

Diagnosis

Usually the diagnosis of bacterial folliculitis is based on the patient's history and clinical presentation. If the diagnosis is unclear or if the folliculitis is not resolving with typical treatment, several tests may be used to discern the etiology. Gram staining is useful in determining the causative organism. Also, a fungal or viral culture can help rule out a non-bacterial cause or rule in dermatophytic folliculitis or herpes folliculitis.

Oftentimes a culture is performed and the result returns as "culture-negative" which is also referred to as "sterile folliculitis". Not all cases of folliculitis are infectious. It can also be caused by irritation from shaving, perspiration, friction, and occlusion in intertriginous areas. In fact, many cases of sterile folliculitis are diagnosed in young, athletic men who perspire every day. Other potential risk factors for this type of folliculitis include poor hygiene, obesity, and diabetes.

Chemicals can also irritate the skin and cause folliculitis. This is often seen with tar-based products and mineral oil. Other chemicals that can cause inflammation of the hair follicle are systemic medications. Chronic use of corticosteroids are infamous for causing "steroid folliculitis" of the face and back. Other triggers include androgens, anti-convulsants, and isotretinoin, which affect the face. A study by Kalapurakal et al. demonstrated that epidermal growth factor inhibitors (EDGFI) like cetuximab and erlotinib caused an acute acneiform folliculitis in 50–100 % of patients. The result is an acute eruption of folliculitis that is distributed over the shoulders, upper arms, and trunk. This reaction is treated successfully with minocycline, steroids, and cessation of the offending medication. Cysts and adnexal tumors also present as subcutaneous lesions. Microscopic examination can easily distinguish this from the other.

Acne keloidalis is a type of folliculitis found commonly in black males at the posterior nape of their neck. Microscopically, the hair follicles are ruptured which results in a dense inflammatory infiltrate and marked fibrous surrounding the area. Free hair shafts are seen eliciting a foreign body giant cell response.

Treatment

In most cases, mild folliculitis heals spontaneously without any sign of scarring. Topical mupirocin can be used in these patients. Scarring or post inflammatory hyperpigmentation may occur if the infection deepens or if the patient excoriates the affected areas. Furunculosis can occur if the *Staphylococcus* infection spreads into the deeper part of the hair follicle.

Moderate to severe cases of folliculitis may be treated with systemic antibiotics in addition to topical antibiotics. For

MSSA, cephalexin or dicloxacillin are recommended. In cases of MRSA doxycycline and TMP-SMX both work well. *Pseudomonas* responds well to ciprofloxacin. For patients who are symptomatic but culture-negative, benzoyl peroxide, topical clindamycin, and an oral tetracycline are recommended. Pruritus may be treated with a short term, low dose of hydrocortisone. A novel formulation that consists of plant extracts has been shown to exhibit potent anti-microbial activity against a broad spectrum of Gram positive and negative organisms, including MRSA.

Prevention

The key to preventing folliculitis lies in establishing good personal hygiene habits, avoiding contaminated hot tubs, frequently replacing razor blades, and if diabetic, maintaining good glucose control.

Recommended Reading

Bolognia JL. Folliculitis and other follicular disorders. Dermatology. Jorizzo JL, Schaffer JV, editors. 3rd ed. N.p.: Waltham: Elsevier; 2012. p. 571–86. Print.

Cohen PR. Community-acquired methicillin-resistant Staphylococcus aureus infections: implications for patients and practitioners. Am J Clin Dermatol. 2007;8(5):259–70.

Eng W, Norman R. Development of an oregano-based ointment with anti-microbial activity including activity against methicillin-resistant Staphylococcus aureus. J Drugs Dermatol. 2010;9(4):377–80.

Kalapurakal SJ, Malone J, Robbins KT, Buescher L, Godwin J, Rao K. Cetuximab in refractory skin cancer treatment. J Cancer. 2012;3:257–61.

Luelmo-Aguilar J, Santandreu MS. Folliculitis: recognition and management. Am J Clin Dermatol. 2004;5(5):301–10.

Lutz JK, Lee J. Prevalence and antimicrobial-resistance of Pseudomonas aerguinosa in swimming pools and hot tubs. Int J Environ Res Public Health. 2011;8(2):554–64.

Case 17
50 Year Old Male with Confluent, Scaly Plaque Covering the Inguinal Area and Extending to Both Inner Thighs

William Eng and Martin J. Walsh

History and Clinical

A 50-year-old male presented for an evaluation for painful lesions found on his interior thigh and groin. The patient stated that he had been hospitalized and had surgical excisions for these lesions, but they had not completely resolved. The patient had no known drug related allergies; he had a history of hypertension.

W. Eng, MD (✉)
Department of Pathology,
University of Central Florida Medical School, Orlando, FL, USA
e-mail: drwilliameng@yahoo.com

M.J. Walsh, MS, BA
Graduate Studies, USF College of Medicine, Tampa, FL, USA

R.A. Norman, W. Eng (eds.), *Clinical Cases in Infections and Infestations of the Skin*, Clinical Cases in Dermatology 6, DOI 10.1007/978-3-319-14295-1_17, © Springer International Publishing Switzerland 2015

Physical Examination

A skin examination showed a slightly scaly plaque in the inguinal area (Fig. 17.1). The patient also complained to have a persistent pruritis and inflammation on his scalp.

Clinical Differential Diagnosis

• Tinea versicolor
• Inverse psoriasis
• Candidiasis
• Erythrasma

Histopathology

A shave biopsy of the outer groin was performed which measured 0.7×0.3×0.1 cm (Specimen A). The Periodic Acid-Schiff stain tested negative for fungus. Filamentous bacteria were seen in the stratum corneum (Fig. 17.2).

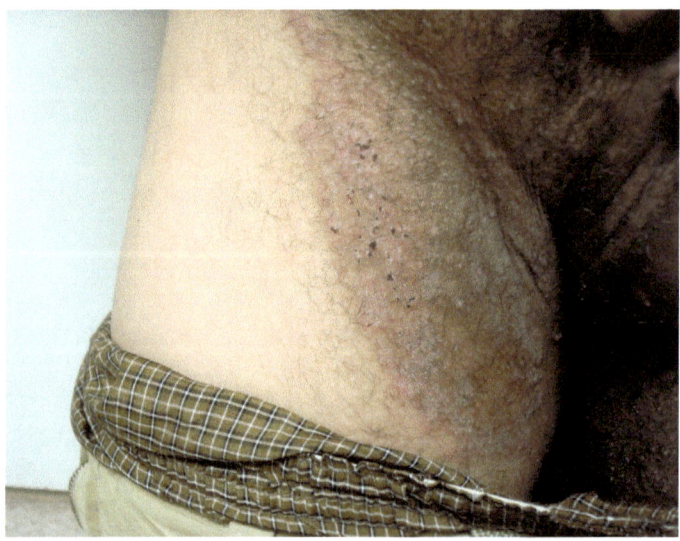

FIGURE 17.1 Erythrasma

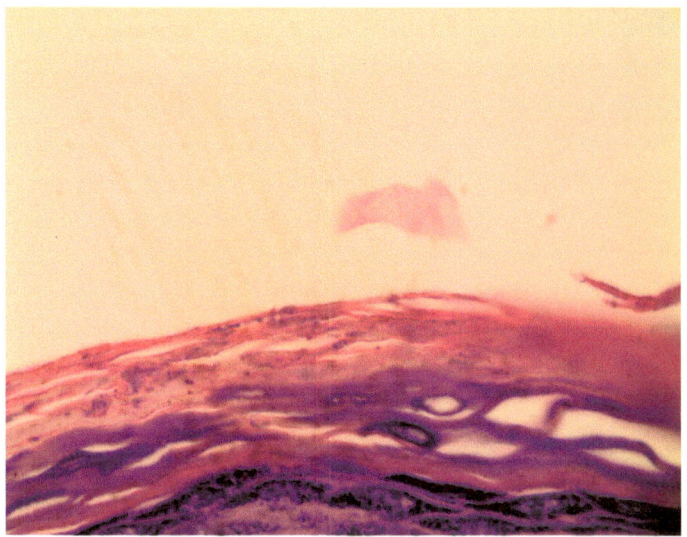

FIGURE 17.2 H&E 1,000×, erythrasma, numerous rod shaped bacteria are seen

Diagnosis

ERYTHRASMA. This disorder is caused by the filamentous bacteria, Corynebacterium minutissimum. Another common site of infection is the toe web between the four and fifth toes. In this area, it presents as a hyperkeratotic yellowish area. Examination by Woods light reveals a coral-red fluorescence of the scales due to porphyrin production by the bacteria.

Treatment Options

This lesion was treated with Drysol 20 % topical solution, Zeasorb-AF 2 % topical powder and was recommended twice daily application to the groin area. Other treatments include Benzoyl peroxide 5 % wash, Clindamycin or Erythromycin or azole creams.

Recommended Reading

Goldsmith LA. Fitzpatrick's dermatology in general medicine. 8th ed. New York: McGraw-Hill Co; 2012. p. 2146–47.

Case 18
27 Year Old Black Male with a Widespread Recurrent Rash Which Occasionally Forms Vesicles

William Eng and Martin J. Walsh

History and Clinical

A 27-year-old African-American male presented with a recurring rash which occasionally forms vesicular lesions containing clear fluid. The lesions were pruritic and spread over much of the skin surface. The patient had been given Bactrim-400 mg oral tablets, but the lesions failed to resolve. The patient had a history and treatment of syphilis, was diagnosed as HIV positive and no reported sexual contact.

———

W. Eng, MD (✉)
Department of Pathology,
University of Central Florida Medical School, Orlando, FL, USA
e-mail: drwilliameng@yahoo.com

M.J. Walsh, MS, BA
Graduate Studies, USF College of Medicine, Tampa, FL, USA

R.A. Norman, W. Eng (eds.), *Clinical Cases in Infections and Infestations of the Skin*, Clinical Cases in Dermatology 6, DOI 10.1007/978-3-319-14295-1_18,
© Springer International Publishing Switzerland 2015

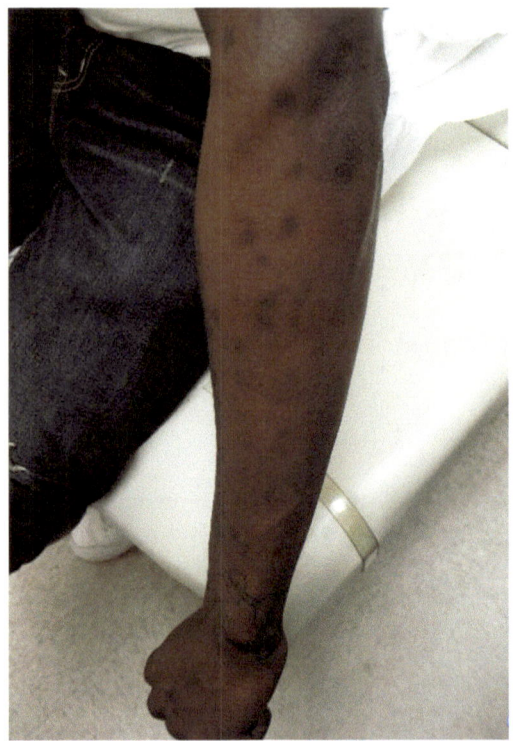

FIGURE 18.1 Syphilis, left lower arm

Physical Examination

The patient had a normal appearance, no distress, and strong acute alertness. Inspection of the skin revealed multiple lesions that consisted of macules and patches of hyperpigmented skin (Figs. 18.1, 18.2, and 18.3).

Clinical Differential Diagnosis

- Drug eruption
- Allergic dermatitis
- Syphilis
- Lichenoid dermatitis

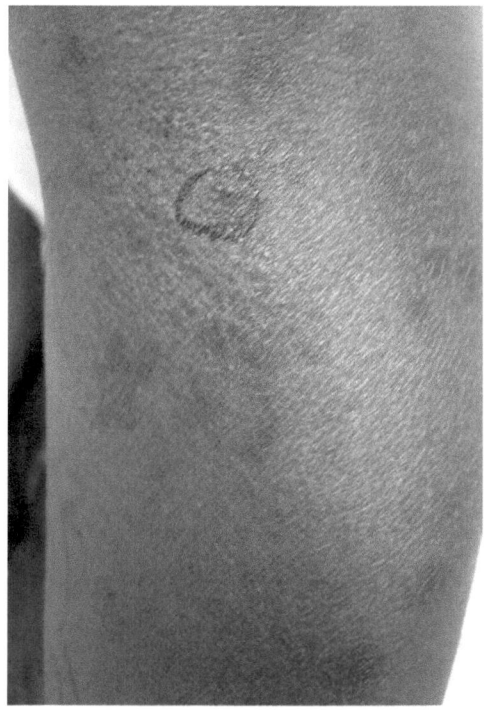

FIGURE 18.2 Syphilis, small dark, vesicular lesions on the median of the patient's left leg

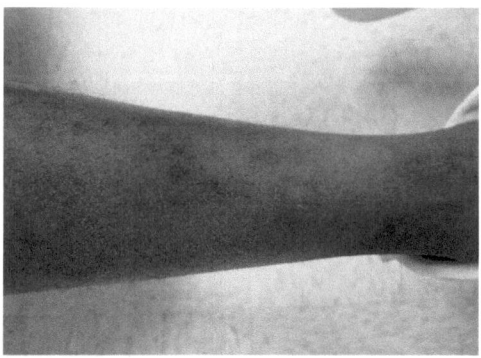

FIGURE 18.3 Syphilis, hyperpigmented patches found throughout the lower extremities

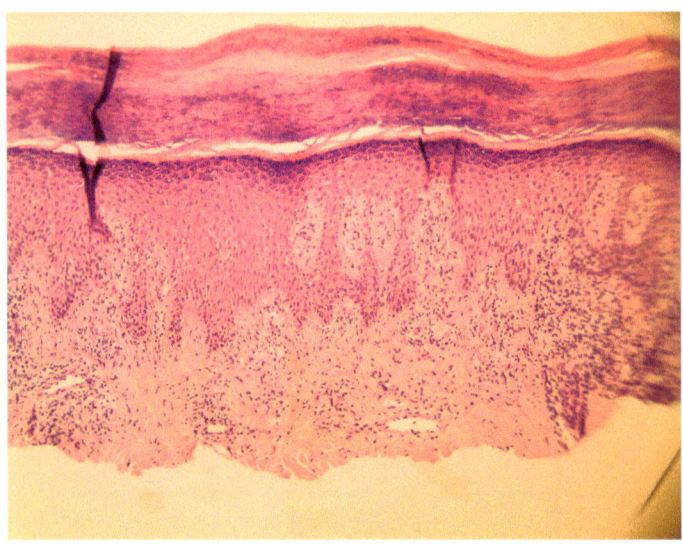

FIGURE 18.4 H&E 100×, Syphilis, psoriasiform epidermal changes

Histopathology

A shave biopsy was performed on the superior left arm (Fig. 18.1), and the medial left leg (Figs. 18.2 and 18.3) and both specimens measured about 0.6×0.5×0.1 cm. The low magnification showed a psoriasiform epidermal pattern with a chronic inflammatory infiltrate (Fig. 18.4). Sections showed a dense, interstitial infiltrate of lymphocytes and numerous plasma cells at high magnification (Fig. 18.5). An immunostain for spirochetes revealed numerous, short-rod shaped organisms in the lower epidermis and upper dermis (Fig. 18.6). Only at higher magnification, the corkscrew form of the spirochetes were appreciated (Fig. 18.7).

Diagnosis

SYPHILIS. This infection is caused by Treponema palladium which is a motile spiral shaped bacteria. It is unique in that it cannot be cultured due to its metabolic requirements. It clini-

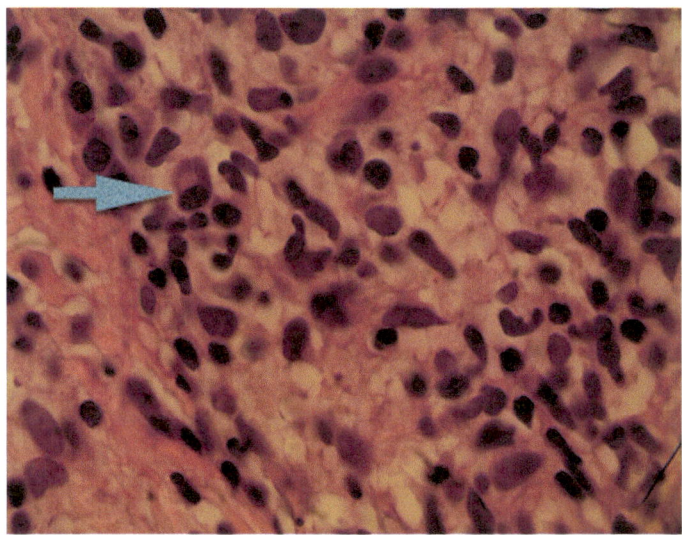

FIGURE 18.5 H&E 1,000×, syphilis, characteristic infiltrate of plasma cells (*arrow*) mixed with lymphocytes

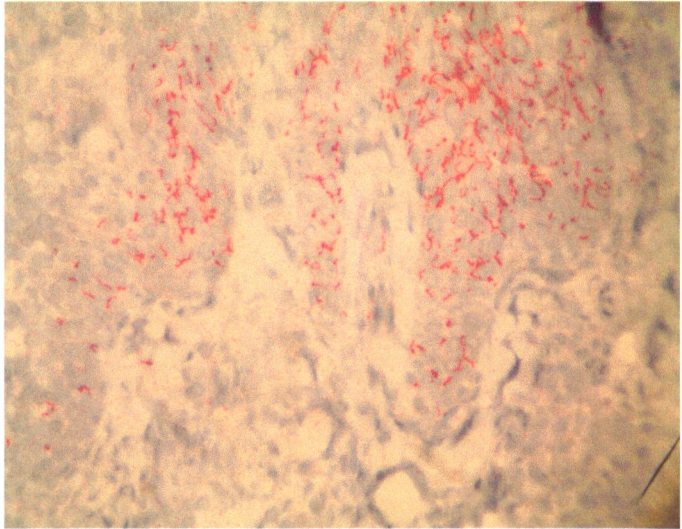

FIGURE 18.6 Syphilis immunostain 400×, numerous spirochetes staining red are found within the lower epidermis

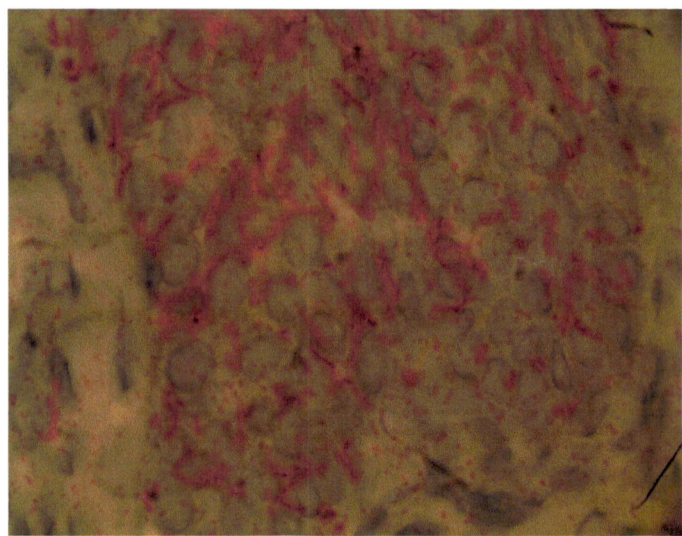

FIGURE 18.7 Syphilis immunostain 1,000×, showing corkscrew organisms

cal appearance can be highly variable, hence it has been called the Great Masquerader/Imitator/Mimic. Lesions can appear ulcerated, lichenoid, macular, papulosquamous, annular, papular, plaques. Secondary syphilis appears on the acral surfaces of the hands and feet as hyperpigmented round macules (copper penny sign). Syphilis can infect an unborn child via trans-placental mode (TORCH infection).

Both a drug eruption and an allergic reaction would elicit eosinophils which are not found in this case. Lichenoid dermatitis would show a lichenoid band of lymphocytes with interface changes which is not seen either. Microscopically, other psoriasiform dermatitis could be in the differential, but the clinical history and immunostaining finding would help lead to the correct diagnosis.

Treatment

- Penicillin G

Recommended Reading

Goldsmith LA. Fitzpatrick's dermatology in general medicine. 8th ed. New York: McGraw-Hill Co; 2012. p. 2471–92.

Part III
Fungal

Case 19
48 Year Old HIV + Male with Multiple Papules and Nodules on Arms

William Eng and Lisa M. Diaz

History and Clinical

A HIV positive 48 year old male presented with multiple papules and nodules on his arms. He reported having chest pain and a non-productive cough. He reported recently having explored several caves with his friends in eastern Tennessee.

Physical Examination

The patient was covered with multiple flesh colored papules and nodules that was neither painful nor pruritic. They had been slowly growing since he came back from his caving trip. The patient had recently developed a low grade fever.

W. Eng, MD (✉)
Department of Pathology,
University of Central Florida Medical School, Orlando, FL, USA
e-mail: drwilliameng@yahoo.com

L.M. Diaz, DO
Lake Erie College of Osteopathic Medicine, Bradenton, FL, USA

R.A. Norman, W. Eng (eds.), *Clinical Cases in Infections and Infestations of the Skin*, Clinical Cases in Dermatology 6, DOI 10.1007/978-3-319-14295-1_19,
© Springer International Publishing Switzerland 2015

Clinical Differential Diagnosis

- Molloscum contagiosum
- Histoplasmosis
- Warts
- Keratoacanthoma

Diagnosis

HISTOPLASMOSIS is an infection caused by the dimorphic fungus *Histoplasma capsulatum.* It is also referred to as Ohio Valley disease, Darling's disease or cave disease. There are two clinical variants: var *capsulatum* and var *duboisii*. It has been divided into three clinical forms: acute pulmonary, chronic cavitary, and disseminated disease. The most common organ involved is the lung, followed by the spleen and the liver. Due to the myriad of clinical presentations that it can assume, histoplasmosis has been deemed the "fungal syphilis." Most cases of histoplasmosis in immunocompetent individuals are asymptomatic and self-limiting. In cases of immunocompromised hosts, disseminated disease may occur in which cutaneous involvement is likely to appear. It is considered an AIDS-defining illness and is generally only seen in patients with CD4 counts of less than 150 cells/mm^3.

Cutaneous histoplasmosis usually occurs on the face, arms, or upper chest and may present as molluscum-like papules, plaques, nodules, or ulcerating lesions. These ulcers may involve the gastrointestinal tract including the tongue, gums, lips, pharynx, and larynx. Histoplasmosis may also present in the form of erythema nodosum, erythema multiforme, pyoderma gangrenosum, panniculitis, abscesses or cellulitis. The disease usually spreads hematogenously but there are rare cases reported of direct inoculation.

The *capsulatum* variant of histoplasmosis is usually found in the Ohio or Mississippi river valleys and the surrounding areas. The *duboisii* variant, also referred to as the African variant, is endemic to Central and Western Africa. The infection occurs when spores found in dried soil, bird or bat droppings are inhaled and travel to the bronchioles of the lungs where they establish a primary infection complex that can then spread to the spleen and liver.

The diagnosis of histoplasmosis can be made with biopsy and direct microscopy. This option is preferred because if the diagnosis is made, treatment can be initiated immediately. On microscopic exam, granulomas can be seen with or without caseating necrosis (Figs. 19.1 and 19.2). The presence of narrow-based budding yeasts can be observed inside or outside of macrophages (Fig. 19.3). The gold standard for diagnosis is culture of the skin lesion. Cultures may also be performed on blood, sputum, bone marrow, lymph nodes or the liver. Fungal growth is extremely slow and culture plates must be kept for 12 weeks. Because histoplasmosis is considered an AIDS-defining illness, HIV testing should

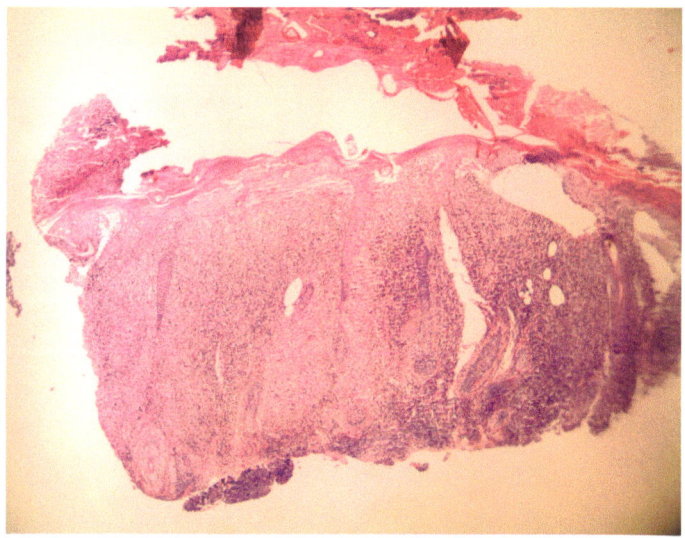

FIGURE 19.1 H&E 40×, Histoplasmosis, most of the entire punch biopsy specimen contains dense inflammation

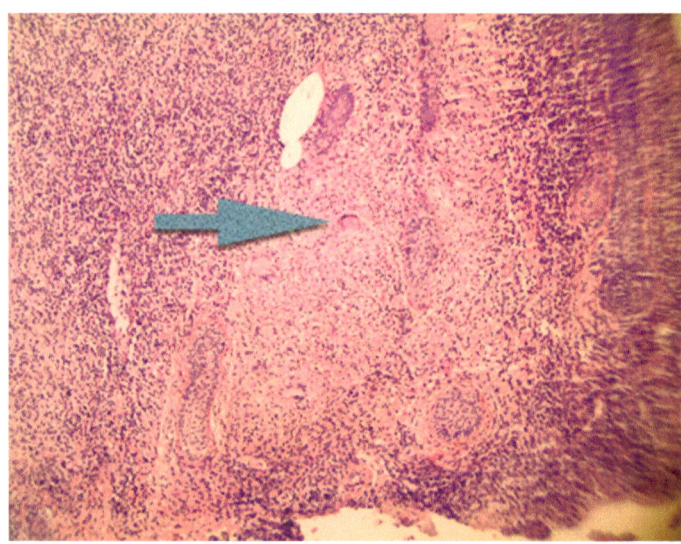

FIGURE 19.2 H&E 100×, Histoplasmosis, confluent granulomas with scattered giant cells (*arrow*)

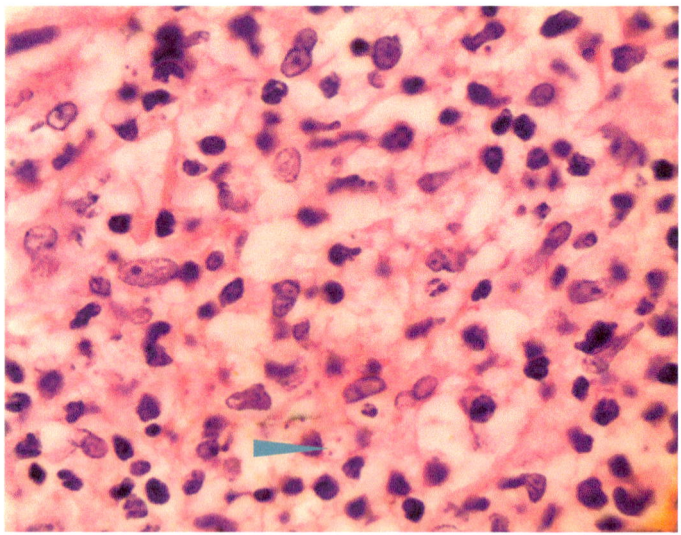

FIGURE 19.3 H&E 1,000×, Histoplasmosis, numerous small dot-like organisms are seen between cells (*arrow*)

be performed in all patients presenting with the disease. Also, imaging studies may be used to check for disseminated disease. Antigen detection provides a rapid test for diagnosis in cases of disseminated disease and may be used to track treatment response.

The clinical appearance of multiple, small dome-shaped lesions such as warts, molloscum, and keratoacanthomas can be distinguished by microscopic examination which shows characteristic histoplasma organisms on routine H&E stains.

Treatment Options

Depending on the severity of disease and the immune status of the patient, itraconazole 200–400 mg daily is recommended. For patients with moderate to severe disease, amphotericin B (1 mg/kg IV daily) is used in combination with itraconazole.

A study by Ramos-e-Silva et al. recommended prophylactic 200 mg itraconazole therapy daily for patients who were HIV positive with CD4 cell counts less than 100–150/mm^3 and who live or have lived near endemic areas. They recommended stopping therapy if the patient became asymptomatic, had improved immune status on anti-retroviral therapy for 6 months, or if there was an undetectable viral load with a CD4 count greater than 150 cells/mm^3. The study found that there was a 95 % mortality rate in cases of untreated disseminated histoplasmosis.

Recommended Reading

Chang P, Rodas C. Skin lesions in histoplasmosis. Clin Dermatol. 2012;30(6):592–8.

Ezzedine K, Accoceberry I, Malvy D. Oral histoplasmosis after radiation therapy for laryngeal squamous cell carcinoma. J Am Acad Dermatol. 2007;56(5):871–3.

Lebwohl MG, Heymann WR, John BJ, Ian C. "Histoplasmosis." Treatment of skin disease: comprehensive therapeutic strategies. 4th ed. Waltham: Elsevier Limited; 2014. p. 316–18.

Ramos-e-Silva M, Oliveira Lima CM, Schechtman RC, Trope BM, Carneiro S. Systemic mycoses in immunodepressed patients (AIDS). Clin Dermatol. 2012;30(6):616–27.

Rodriguez-Cerdeira C, Arenas R, Moreno-Coutino G, Vazquez E, Fernandez R, Chang P. Systemic fungal infections in patients with human immunodeficiency virus. Actas Dermosifiliogr. 2014;105(1):5–17.

Case 20
32 Year Old Female with Thickened, Yellowish, Friable Fingernails and Toenails

William Eng and Martin J. Walsh

History and Clinical

A 32-year-old female presented with a complaint that her nails were constantly breaking.

Physical Examination

The patient's fingernails showed hyperkeratosis with a yellowish hue. The edges were irregular and friable (Fig. 20.1) and under the nail, loose fragments of cornified debris were found.

W. Eng, MD (✉)
Department of Pathology,
University of Central Florida Medical School, Orlando, FL, USA
e-mail: drwilliameng@yahoo.com

M.J. Walsh, MS, BA
Graduate Studies, USF College of Medicine, Tampa, FL, USA

R.A. Norman, W. Eng (eds.), *Clinical Cases in Infections and Infestations of the Skin*, Clinical Cases in Dermatology 6, DOI 10.1007/978-3-319-14295-1_20, © Springer International Publishing Switzerland 2015

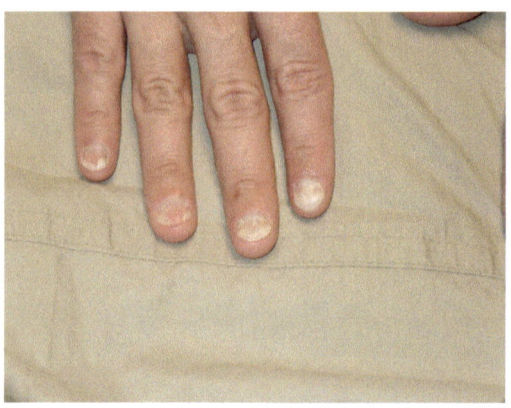

FIGURE 20.1 Onychomycosis of fingernails

Clinical Differential Diagnosis

(Friable nail)

* Psoriatic nail
* Bacteria infection
* Fungal/Yeast infection
* Mixed fungal and bacteria infection
* Lichen planus
* Pachyonchia Congenita

Histopathology

The nail clipping was sectioned and measured at $0.5 \times 0.2 \times 0.1$ cm. The Gram stains showed gram-positive cocci. The PAS stain showed branching, septated hyphae (Fig. 20.2).

Diagnosis

ONYCHOMYCOSIS WITH BACTERIA INFECTION OF THE NAIL. Fungal infection of the nail is found in up to 14 % of the population. Common risk factors include nail trauma, HIV infection, diabetes mellitus, peripheral vascular

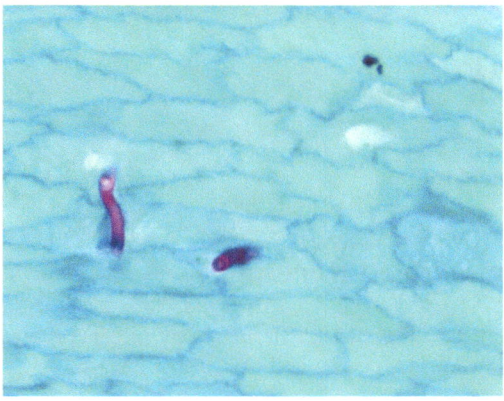

FIGURE 20.2 PAS stain 1,000×, Fungal hyphae (*red*) are found within the nail plate

disease. Around 30–40 % of the patients with nail fungus infection also have a concomitant fungal infection of the skin, particularly of the foot. The two most common toenail dermatophytes involved are T. rubum and T. interdigitate which account for 90 % of all cases. Yeast and molds account for the remaining 10 %. However, yeasts account for 30 % of fingernail infections. Three clinical patterns have been described-distolateral subungal, proximal subungual (T. rubrum and megninii), and superficial white type (T. interdigitale).

Psoriasis of the nail can result in yellowish discoloration (oil spot) while lichen planus can have a brown discoloration with friable changes and pitting. Pachyonchia congenita is an autosomal dominant malformation of the nail. However, a fungus stain (PAS or GMS) would be negative in these cases.

Treatment Options

Topical

- Ketoconazole
- Ciclopirox
- Amorolfine

Systemic

- Terbinafine
- Itraconazole
- Fluconazole

Surgical removal

Recommended Reading

Goldsmith LA. Fitzpatrick's dermatology in general medicine. 8th ed. New York: McGraw-Hill Co; 2012. p. 2292–6.

Case 21
49 Year Old White Female with Pigmented Lesions on Chest

William Eng and Martin J. Walsh

History and Clinical

A 49-year-old female presented with brownish-red lesions on her chest that had been morphologically changing over the past 4 months. She also requested that several skin growths be removed as they had been bothersome over the past 5 years. The patient was taking the following medications at time of service: Mupirocin 2 % topical cream, Cephalexin 500 mg oral capsule.

Physical Examination

Patient appeared normal in mood, affect and presented as healthy. Her sternal regions showed maculopapular brown lesions. The patient had bilateral 2–3 cm, irregular border, bi-colored nevi on the superior and inferior aspects of both her breasts (Fig. 21.1).

———
W. Eng, MD (✉)
Department of Pathology, University of Central Florida Medical School, Orlando, FL, USA
e-mail: drwilliameng@yahoo.com

M.J. Walsh, MS, BA
Graduate Studies, USF College of Medicine, Tampa, FL, USA

R.A. Norman, W. Eng (eds.), *Clinical Cases in Infections and Infestations of the Skin*, Clinical Cases in Dermatology 6, DOI 10.1007/978-3-319-14295-1_21,
© Springer International Publishing Switzerland 2015

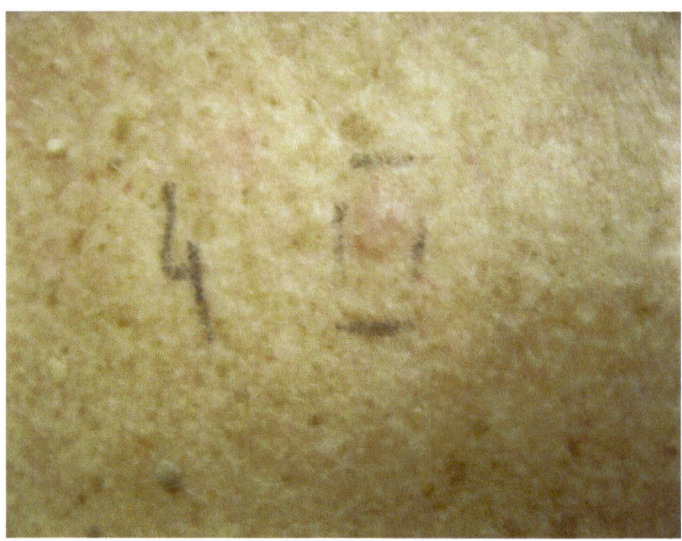

FIGURE 21.1 Compound dysplastic nevus, *brownish-red* papule on right breast

Clinical Differential Diagnosis

- Nevus
- Lentigo
- Macular seborrheic keratosis
- Post inflammatory hyperpigmentation
- Compound dysplastic nevus with yeast (Pityrosporum)

Histopathology

Sections showed junctional and dermal melanocytic nests. No inflammatory cells were found within the dermis. The cornified layer showed numerous round organisms at the follicular opening (Figs. 21.2 and 21.3).

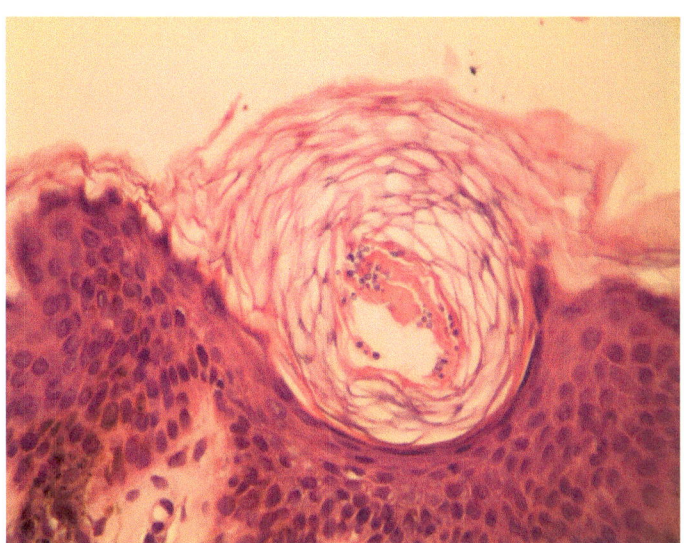

FIGURE 21.2 H&E 400×, Pityrosporum yeasts at the follicular osmium

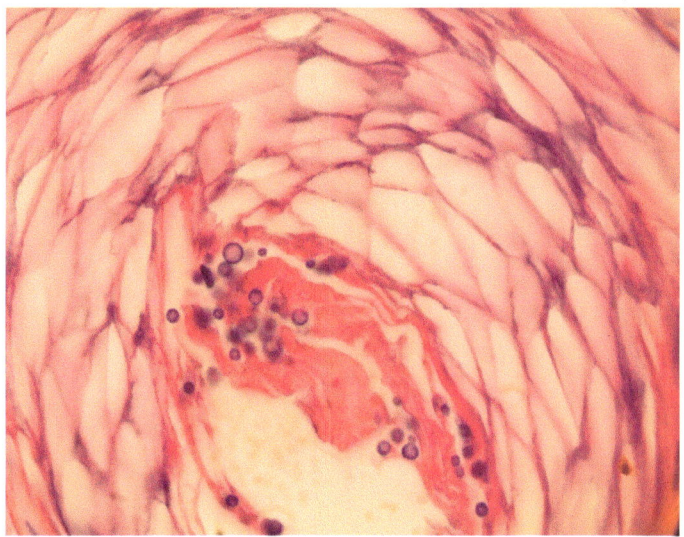

FIGURE 21.3 H&E 1,000×, Pityrosporum yeast, multiple round organisms found only with the cornified layer

Diagnosis

PITYROSPORUM YEAST (in a compound dysplastic nevus with mild atypia). There are 12 known species of this yeast malassezia fur fur, pachydermatis, sykpodialis, globosa, restricta, slooffiae, obtuse, dermatitis, nana, yamatoensis, japonica and equi. All require lipid for growth. It is the etiology of two infectious processes, Pityriasis vesicular and Pityriasis folliculitis. They also play a role in seborrheic dermatitis, atopic dermatitis, and psoriasis. These organisms are commonly found around the face, and co-exists in a symbiotic relationship without causing disease.

The differential of a pigmented lesion can include a nevus which would show a population of nevus cells at the junction or in the dermis. A lentigo, however, would have an increase of melanocytes along the junction with increased pigmentation of the basal keratinocytes, but no nevus nests in the dermis. Post inflammatory hyperpigmentation will exhibit free melanin pigment in the superficial dermis, but no increase of melanocyte. A macular seborrheic keratosis also does not show an increase of melanocytes, only a thickening of the epidermis.

Treatment Options

- None- if no pathological disease is present
- Ketoconazole

Recommended Reading

Goldsmith LA et al. Fitzpatrick's dermatology in general medicine. 8th ed. New York: McGraw-Hill Co; 2012. p. 2307–9.

Case 22
56 Year Old with a Widespread, Slightly Itchy Rash with Discoloration

William Eng and Martin J. Walsh

History and Clinical

A 56 female presented at the clinic complaining of a widespread rash. The rash was mildly itchy and becomes prominent when exposed to sunlight and after showering.

Physical Exam

The patient showed multiple round to oval hypo-pigmented flat lesions. A small amount of overlying scale was noted in some of the lesions (Fig. 22.1).

W. Eng, MD (✉)
Department of Pathology, University of Central Florida Medical School, Orlando, FL, USA
e-mail: drwilliameng@yahoo.com

M.J. Walsh, MS, BA
Graduate Studies, USF College of Medicine, Tampa, FL, USA

R.A. Norman, W. Eng (eds.), *Clinical Cases in Infections and Infestations of the Skin*, Clinical Cases in Dermatology 6, DOI 10.1007/978-3-319-14295-1_22,
© Springer International Publishing Switzerland 2015

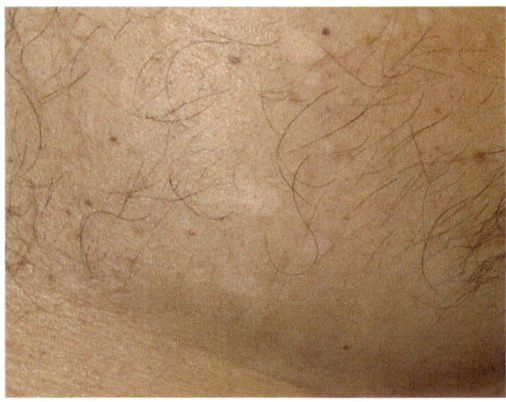

FIGURE 22.1   Tinea versicolor, hypopigmented round-oval flat lesions

Clinical Differential Diagnosis

(Pigmentation changes with minimal erythema)

- Vitiligo
- Post inflammatory hypopigmentation
- Idiopathic guttate hypomelanosis
- Tinea versicolor

Histopathology

Sections showed minimal inflammation in the dermis. Within the cornified layer, numerous small yeast like organisms and hyphae structures were found by routine H&E (Fig. 22.2) or by KOH skin scraping prep (Fig. 22.3).

Diagnosis

TINEA VERSICOLOR. This is one of the most common dermatological disorders seen. The causative agent is usually Malassezia furfur which is a dimorphic, lipophilic organism

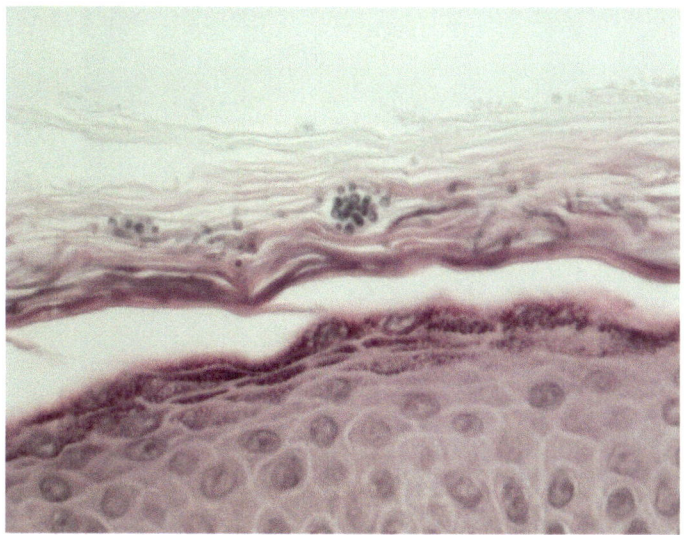

FIGURE 22.2 H&E 400×, Tinea versicolor showing numerous fungal yeast and hyphae forms found in the cornified layer

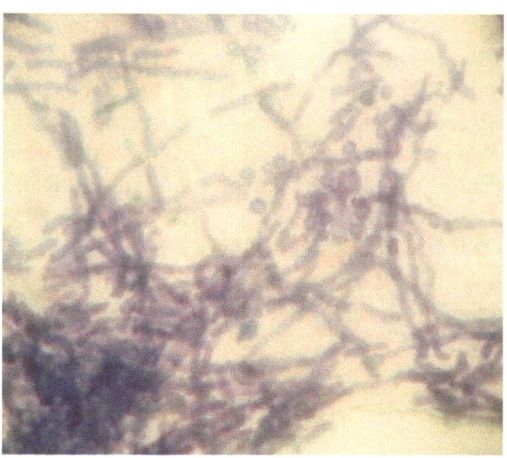

FIGURE 22.3 KOH prep 1,000×, Tinea versicolor showing numerous fungal hyphae and yeast forms

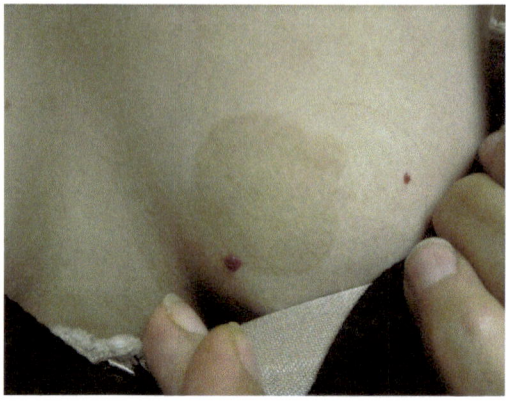

FIGURE 22.4 Tinea versicolor, hyperpigmented patches with two incidental hemangiomas on the breast

which converts from a yeast form to a parasitic mycelial form. This transformation is stimulated by a warm, humid environment, hyperhidrosis, steroids, Cushing's disease, immunosuppression, and a malnourished state. The yeast filters natural sunlight leading to zones of hypo-pigmentation. However, in some patients it may appear as hyper-pigmented (Fig. 22.4). Re-infection is common, so the patient needs to be instructed in cleaning all articles of clothing, bed, chairs and other areas where contact with the skin can lead to re-infection.

Pigmentation changes can be similar clinically, but on microscopic examination, the fungal elements are easily identified residing within the cornified layer. MART-1 immunostain along with a Fontana Masson stain can be helpful categorizing the basis of the pigmentation changes.

Treatment Options

- Ketoconazole
- Fluconazole
- Itraconazole

Recommended Reading

Goldsmith LA et al. Fitzpatrick's dermatology in general medicine. 8th ed. New York: McGraw-Hill Co; 2012. p. 2307–9.

Case 23
46 Year Old Female with a Rapidly Spreading Rash

William Eng and Martin J. Walsh

History and Clinical

A 46 year old female presented with a rapidly spreading rash. She has one pet dog at home.

Physical Exam

One acral hand surface showed diffuse scaling while the other surface has a normal appearance (Fig. 23.1). In areas on the body, the rash appeared round to oval with a scaly center. The edge was slightly keratotic and erythematous (Fig. 23.2). Other areas showed only a vague round lesion (Fig. 23.3).

W. Eng, MD (✉)
Department of Pathology, University of Central Florida Medical School, Orlando, FL, USA
e-mail: drwilliameng@yahoo.com

M.J. Walsh, MS, BA
Graduate Studies, USF College of Medicine, Tampa, FL, USA

R.A. Norman, W. Eng (eds.), *Clinical Cases in Infections and Infestations of the Skin*, Clinical Cases in Dermatology 6, DOI 10.1007/978-3-319-14295-1_23,
© Springer International Publishing Switzerland 2015

127

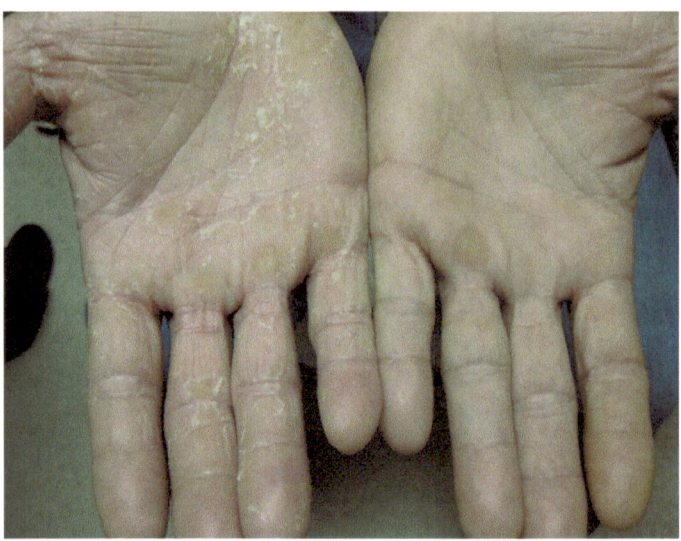

FIGURE 23.1 Tinea corporis (one hand, two feet sign), the palm of the hand and both the bottom of the feet are scaly

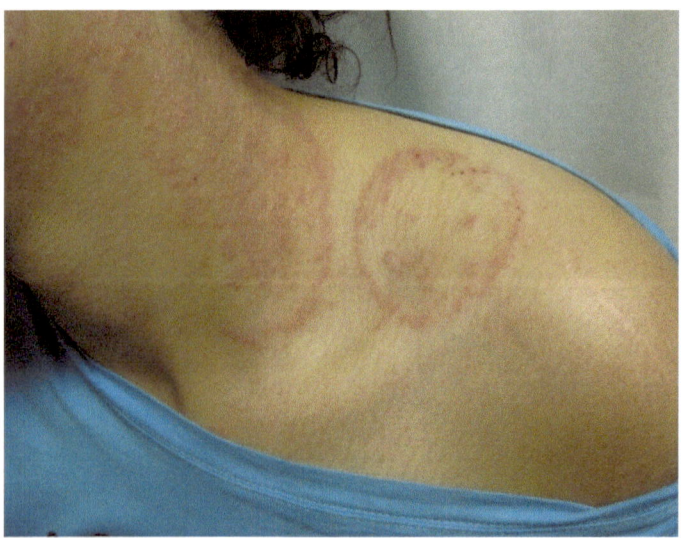

FIGURE 23.2 Tinea corporis, multiple round/oval rash with an active erythematous, scaly outer ring

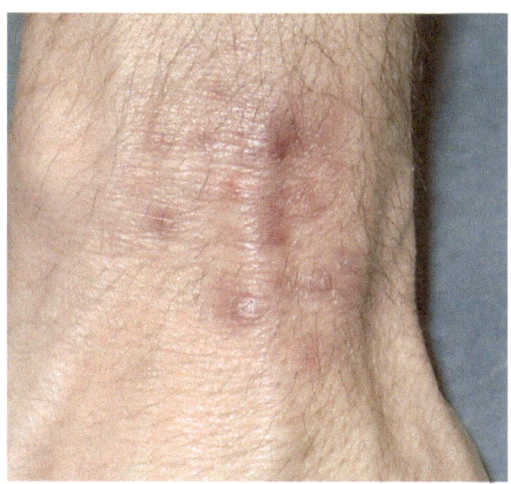

FIGURE 23.3 Tinea corporis-subtype (Mahjocchi's granuloma), vague annular pattern of coalesced papules. The fungus infection spreads along the follicle into the subcutaneous tissue

Clinical Differential Diagnosis

(Annular Rash)

- Contact dermatitis
- Mycosis fungoides
- Tinea corporis (ringworm)
- Subacute lupus erythromatous
- Erythema annular centrifugum
- Nummular eczema
- Candidiasis
- Pityriasis rosea

Histopathology

Sections showed staggered parakeratosis intermingled with fungal hyphae (Fig. 23.4). The dermis showed a mild to moderate perivascular inflammatory infiltrate.

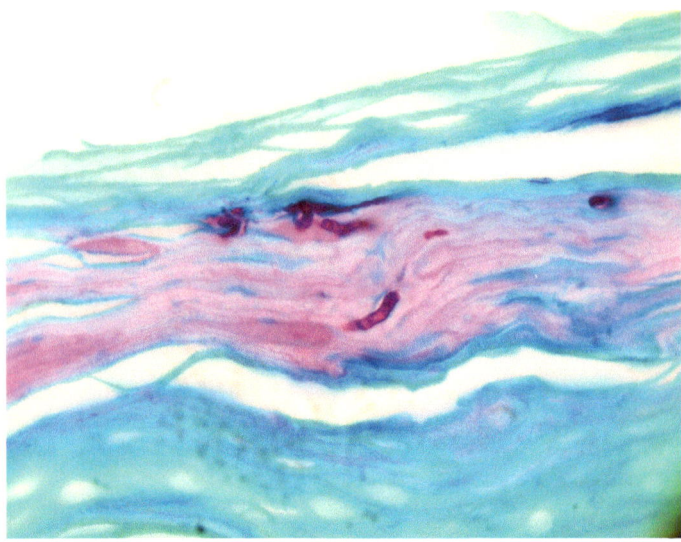

FIGURE 23.4 PAS stain 400×, fungal hyphae is seen within the cornified layer

Diagnosis

TINEA CORPORIS (RINGWORM) This disease is commonly transmitted directly between infected individuals and/or animals. Warm, humid environments also contributes to susceptibility of infection. The most common causative type is T. rubrum. Majocchi's granuloma is used when fungal infection involves the subcutaneous tissue. Identification of the species can be made by observation of the fungal growth on the media plate and by microscopic examination of the fungus and its spores morphology.

A contact dermatitis and nummular dermatitis would have more epidermal changes such as spongiosis. Mycosis fungoides would show atypical cerebreform T cells with minimal spongiosis in the epidermis. Lupus would show interface changes. Erythema annular centrifugum shows a tight perivascular lymphocytic infiltrate (coat sleeve). Candidiasis shows mainly yeast organisms by special stains. Pityriasis rosea shows slight spongiosis with focal mounds of parakeratosis and extravasated RBCs.

Treatment Options

- Terbinafine
- Itraconazole
- Fluconazole
- Griseofulvin
- Ketoconazole

Recommended Reading

Goldsmith LA et al. Fitzpatrick's dermatology in general medicine. 8th ed. New York: McGraw-Hill Co; 2012. p. 2277–97.

Case 24
7 Year Old Male with an Enlarging, Round Area of Hair Loss

William Eng and Martin J. Walsh

History and Clinic

A 7 year old male presented with loss of hair over the past 5 months. It began as a small annular area which slowly enlarged to cover the occipital scalp.

Physical Examination

The child appeared well nourished and developed. There was a discrete loss of hair with a round to oval pattern that was more pronounced at the vertex of the scalp. The scalp itself showed mild erythema and slight scaling (Fig. 24.1).

W. Eng, MD (✉)
Department of Pathology, University of Central Florida Medical School, Orlando, FL, USA
e-mail: drwilliameng@yahoo.com

M.J. Walsh, MS, BA
Graduate Studies, USF College of Medicine, Tampa, FL, USA

R.A. Norman, W. Eng (eds.), *Clinical Cases in Infections and Infestations of the Skin*, Clinical Cases in Dermatology 6, DOI 10.1007/978-3-319-14295-1_24, © Springer International Publishing Switzerland 2015

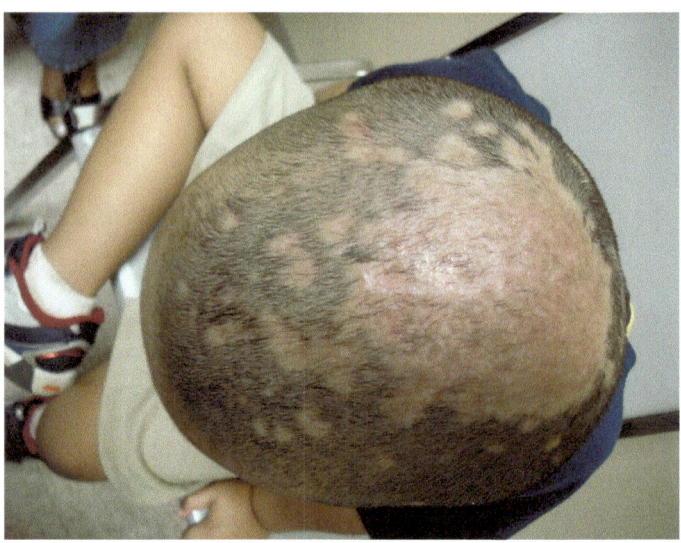

FIGURE 24.1 Tinea capitis, focal and discrete hair loss

Clinical Differential Diagnosis

(Focal Hair Loss)

- Alopecia areta
- Trichotillomania
- Tinea capitis
- Lupus
- Syphilis
- Seborrheic dermatitis
- Bacteria folliculitis

Histopathology

A punch biopsy of the patient's scalp was performed. The biopsy measured 0.2×0.3 cm. The Periodic Acid-Schiff stained numerous hyphae structures within the hair shaft (Fig. 24.2).

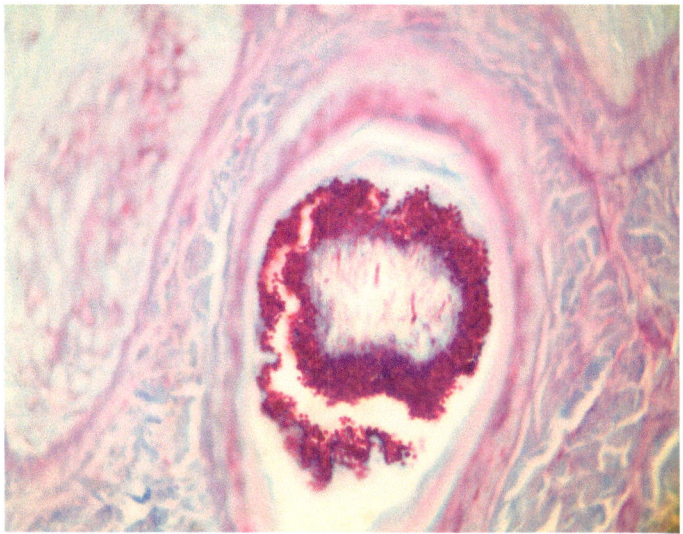

FIGURE 24.2 PAS stain 400×, Numerous fungal organisms involve the hair shaft

Diagnosis

TINEA CAPITIS This infection is caused mainly by either Trichophyton or Microsporum species. It affects children primary between the ages of 3–14.

The differential of focal hair loss should be differentiated from other infections (fungus, bacteria, spirochete, yeast). Appropriate special stains can aid in the identification of these organisms. PAS and GMS stains are used to identify fungal or yeast organisms while Gram or Brown-Bren stains can be used to identify bacteria. A silver stain or immunostain can detect syphilis. An autoimmune etiology, alopecia areata, shows a peribulbar lymphocytic infiltrate (swarm of bees) with a anagen to catagen shift of the follicles.

Treatment Options

- Griseofulvin
- Terbinafine
- Itraconazole
- Fluconazole
- Terbinafine

Recommended Reading

Goldsmith LA et al. Fitzpatrick's dermatology in general medicine. 8th ed. New York: McGraw-Hill Co; 2012. p. 2277–97.

Case 25
76 Year Old Female with Enlarging Painless Nodule on the Arm

William Eng and Lisa M. Diaz

History and Clinical

A 76 year old female presented with an enlarging, painless nodule on her arm. The lesion was slowly enlarging with discharge of putrid pus. She works on her garden in her spare time.

Physical Examination

The arm showed an ill-defined subcutaneous lesion with marked erythema. The area was warm to the touch. Crusted yellowish material was seen coating the surface (Fig. 25.1).

———
W. Eng, MD (✉)
Department of Pathology, University of Central Florida Medical School, Orlando, FL, USA
e-mail: drwilliameng@yahoo.com

L.M. Diaz, DO
Lake Erie College of Osteopathic Medicine,
Bradenton, FL, USA

R.A. Norman, W. Eng (eds.), *Clinical Cases in Infections and Infestations of the Skin*, Clinical Cases in Dermatology 6, DOI 10.1007/978-3-319-14295-1_25,
© Springer International Publishing Switzerland 2015

137

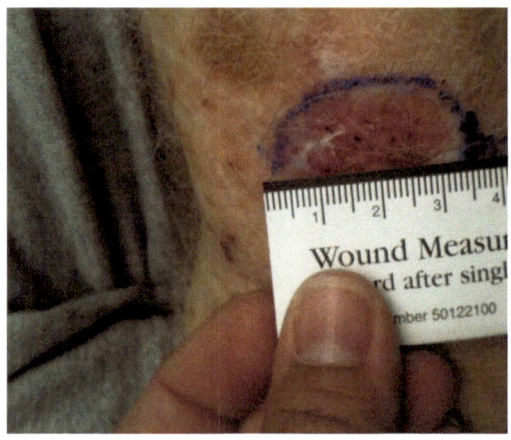

FIGURE 25.1 Chromoblastomycosis infection of the arm

Clinical Differential Diagnosis

- Bacteria abscess
- Fungal infection (Chromoblastomycosis)

Diagnosis

CHROMOBLASTOMYCOSIS is a chronic fungal infection that occurs in the cutaneous and subcutaneous tissues of the lower extremities. It characteristically affects middle-aged men with agricultural occupations in tropical and subtropical climates like Madagascar, Australia, China, Mexico, Cuba, and Africa.

Chromoblastomycosis presents as painless red to violaceous, verrucous papules or plaques with satellite lesions that spread in a centripetal fashion. They are often described as cauliflower-like in appearance. Lesions that have been present for a long time may demonstrate an annular pattern with central clearing. They are usually not painful but can be pruritic and bleed easily when traumatized. Typically only one of the lower extremities is involved but there are cases of upper limb and trunk involvement in non-agricultural areas. One Japanese study of 290 chromoblastomycosis lesions reported that the majority of lesions were found on the upper extremities of men and the faces and necks of women.

Several pigmented (dematiaceous) fungi are responsible for this disease; however *Fonsecaea pedrosoi* is the most common cause and is responsible for more than 80 % of the infections. The other fungi responsible for the remainder of the cases include: *Cladosporium carrionii*, *Fonsecaea compacta*, *Fonsecaea monophora*, *Phialophora verrucosa*, and *Rhinocladiella aquaspersa*. They all produce the characteristic sclerotic bodies (referred to as either Medlar, copper penny or muriform bodies) that can be found intracellularly in macrophages or extracellularly in abscesses.

These fungi are found in soil, plants, and decaying vegetation. Chromoblastomycosis is acquired most commonly by traumatic inoculation. The classic history is an agricultural worker who reports a nodule that formed at the site of a splinter puncture. These lesions usually present 1–2 months after inoculation. Chromoblastomycosis is a slow growing, locally progressive disease that can spread by autoinoculation or through the lymphatic system. Complications of this disease include lymphedema, ulceration, and secondary bacterial infection. Rare cases of malignant transformation to squamous cell carcinoma and melanoma have been reported. These cases occurred after more than 10 years of disease duration.

The diagnosis can be made using direct microscopy, culture, or histopathology. A KOH scraping of the black dots visible on the lesion will demonstrate the characteristic brown sclerotic cells with thick walls that are pathognomonic for chromoblastomycosis (Fig. 25.2). Occasionally dark thick hyphae are identifiable, as well. A culture may then be used to determine the specific fungal species. A biopsy will show a granulomatous lesion with sclerotic bodies and an epidermis that is thickened due to a process known as pseudoepitheliomatous hyperplasia. A host response process referred to as transepithelial elimination occurs when dermal fungi material

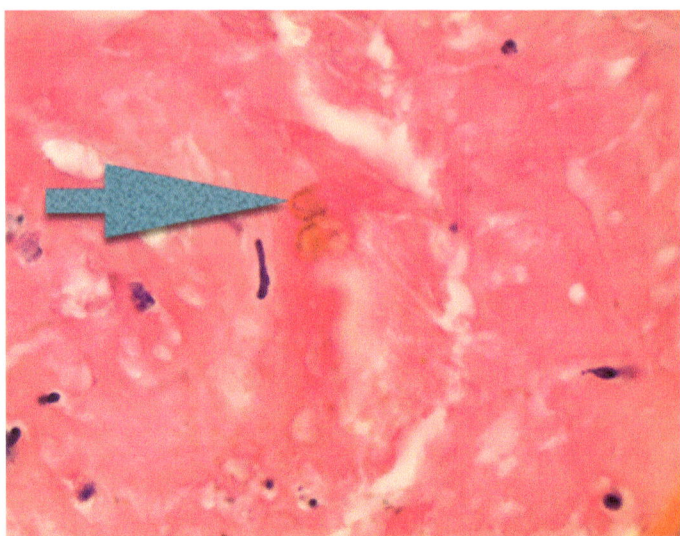

FIGURE 25.2 H&E 1,000×, Chromoblastomycosis (tip of *arrow*) appear as multiple round yellowish-tan "copper penny" organisms

and damaged tissue are expelled through the epidermis. The visible characteristic black dots on the surface of the lesions are the result of this process and represent fungal and necrotic debris.

Treatment

Chromoblastomycosis is difficult to treat and is prone to recurrence especially if the cutaneous involvement is extensive. Cure rates in the literature vary from 15 to 80 %. The success of the treatment is dependent on multiple factors including fungal species, extent of disease, and whether the patient has edema or dermal fibrosis. The most common offender, *F. pedrosoi*, is also the most recalcitrant and difficult to eradicate. *C. carinii and P. verrucosa* are the most sensitive to treatment.

Surgical excision with wide margins can be utilized with small, localized lesions. Chemotherapy is often used after excision to decrease the risk of relapse. Cryosurgery can also be used for treatment and is a less expensive option. High doses of oral antifungals like itraconazole (100–400 mg daily) or terbinafine (250–500 mg daily) can be used alone for therapy or in combination in cases of advanced disease. Oral antifungals can also be combined with other treatment options. For example, pre-treating with oral antifungals for 6–12 months to reduce the lesion size and then using either cryosurgery or surgical excision to destroy the remaining lesions. Curettage and electrodessication is discouraged as there are reports of disease spread after this procedure.

Prevention

Workers in tropical climates should wear proper protective clothing including close-toed shoes. Early diagnosis is crucial for treatment and disease control.

Recommended Reading

Bassas-Vila J, Fuente MJ, Guinovart R, Ferrándiz C. Chromoblastomycosis: Response to combination therapy with cryotherapy and terbinafine. Actas Dermo-Sifiliograficas. 2014; 105(2):196–8.

Bonifaz A, Carrasco-Gerard E, Saúl A. Chromoblastomycosis: clinical and mycologic experience of 51 cases. Mycoses. 2001;44:1–7.

Bonifaz A, Paredes-Solis V, Saul A. Treating chromoblastomycosis with systemic antifungals. Expert Opin Pharmacother. 2004;5:247–54.

Castro LG, Pimentel ER, Lacaz CS. Treatment of chromomycosis by cryosurgery with liquid nitrogen: 15 years' experience. Int J Dermatol. 2003;42:408–12.

Fukushiro R. Chromomycosis in Japan. Int J Dermatol. 1983;22: 221–9.

Gon A, Minelli L. Melanoma in a long-standing lesion of chromoblastomycosis. Int J Dermatol. 2006;45:1331–3.

Lopez Martinez R, Mendez Tovar LJ. Chromoblastomycosis. Clin Dermatol. 2007;25(2):188–94.

Mouchalouat Mde F, Gutierrez Galhardo MC, Zancopé-Oliveira RM, Monteiro Fialho PC, de Oliveira Coelho JM, Silva Tavares PM. Chromoblastomycosis: a clinical and molecular study of 18 cases in Rio de Janeiro, Brazil. Int J Dermatol. 2011;50:981–6.

Paul C, Dupont B, Pialoux G. Chromoblastomycosis with malignant transformation and cutaneous-synovial localization: the potential therapeutic role of itraconazole. J Med Vet Mycol. 1991;29: 313–6.

Queiroz-Telles F, McGinnis MR, Salkin I, Graybill JR. Subcutaneous mycoses. Infect Dis Clin North Am. 2003;17:59–85.

Queiroz-Telles F, Esterre P, Perez-Blanco M, Vitale RG, Salgado CG, Bonifaz A. Chromoblastomycosis: an overview of clinical manifestations, diagnosis and treatment. Med Mycol. 2009;47:3–15.

Case 26
68 Year Old HIV + Male with Multiple Acne-Like Growths on the Chest

William Eng and Martin J. Walsh

History and Clinical

A 68 year old HIV positive male who had not been properly taking his medication presented with multiple growths on his chest.

Physical Examination

Examination revealed a variety of lesions from acne-like pustules to vegetating warty growths to ulcerated infiltrative nodules.

Clinical Differential Diagnosis

- Fungal infection (Cryptococcus)
- Neurofibroma

W. Eng, MD (✉)
Department of Pathology, University of Central Florida Medical School, Orlando, FL, USA
e-mail: drwilliameng@yahoo.com

M.J. Walsh, MS, BA
Graduate Studies, USF College of Medicine, Tampa, FL, USA

R.A. Norman, W. Eng (eds.), *Clinical Cases in Infections and Infestations of the Skin*, Clinical Cases in Dermatology 6, DOI 10.1007/978-3-319-14295-1_26, © Springer International Publishing Switzerland 2015

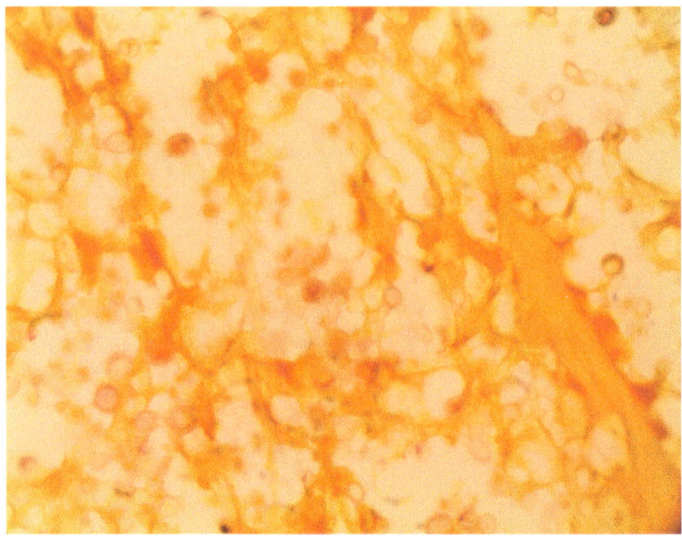

FIGURE 26.I Mucicarmine stain, 1,000×, Cryptococcus neoformis, numerous organisms stain slight reddish with mucoid, thick capsule

- Molloscum
- Tuberous sclerosis

Diagnosis

CRYPTOCOCCUS. The yeast structure measures 5–15 um in diameter, and is surrounded by a thick capsule, typically seen by a mucicarmine stain (Fig. 26.1). While direct examination by India ink continues to be utilized, newer methods of detection are now available which include latex agglutination and ELISA, particularly for CSF.

Cryptococcus is a yeast-like organism that is transmitted by inhalation of infected organisms. Once established, it disseminates to other organs including the skin. Those immunosuppressed such as by HIV infection are particularly susceptible. The prevalence of Cryptococcus infection among the HIV infected has significantly decreased given the increased use of HAART. The most common presentation of infection is meningoencephalitis with altered mental status.

Treatment Options

- Amphotericin B
- Flucytosine
- Fluconazole
- Itraconazole

Recommended Reading

Goldsmith LA et al. Fitzpatrick's dermatology in general medicine. 8th ed. New York: McGraw-Hill Co; 2012. p. 2325–26.

Case 27
56 Year Old Central American Male Immigrant with a Persistent Cough and Chest Pain

William Eng and Lisa M. Diaz

Clinical and History

A 56 year old male who recently immigrated from Equador presented with scattered plaques on his chest.

Physical Examination

In addition to the scattered plaques, the patient also complained of a cough.

W. Eng, MD (✉)
Department of Pathology, University of Central Florida Medical School, Orlando, FL, USA
e-mail: drwilliameng@yahoo.com

L.M. Diaz, DO
College of Osteopathic Medicine, Lake Erie College of Osteopathic Medicine, Bradenton, FL, USA

R.A. Norman, W. Eng (eds.), *Clinical Cases in Infections and Infestations of the Skin*, Clinical Cases in Dermatology 6, DOI 10.1007/978-3-319-14295-1_27,
© Springer International Publishing Switzerland 2015

Clinical Differential Diagnosis

- Cryptococcus
- Chromoblastomycosis
- Histomycosis
- Coccidiomycosis

Diagnosis

COCCIDIOMYCOSIS is a deep fungal infection that is caused by either *Coccidioides immitis* or *C posadasii*. The fungus is endemic to Central Mexico, Central and South America. In the United States, cases have been reported in Arizona and California, which explains the synonym "San Joaquin Valley Fever." The fungus lives in the soil and is transported in the form of spores (arthroconidia) in dust clouds that can then be inhaled by humans. The incidence of coccidioidomycosis is escalating and this trend is attributed to increased development and construction in endemic regions. Most reported cases of coccidioidomycosis occur during the dry season or in times of drought as more dust clouds form and effectively spread spores over farther distances thereby exposing more people to infection.

Coccidioidomycosis may present in many forms. Lesions in disseminated disease may arise via hematogenous or via direct extension from an infected visceral organ, bone, or lymph node. Skin that has lost some protective barrier function, for example in patients with atopic dermatitis, is more likely to develop lesions. Verrucous papules, plaques, and ulcerated lesions are observed most commonly in a patient who presents with disseminated pulmonary disease. Any part of the skin can be affected but sternoclavicular and nasolabial folds are the most commonly seen areas. Toxic erythema is an exanthematous reaction that occurs in approximately 10 % patients immediately after inhalation. It manifests as a generalized pruritic eruption of violaceous papules and plaques, urticarial-like papules, as well as targetoid purpuric papules.

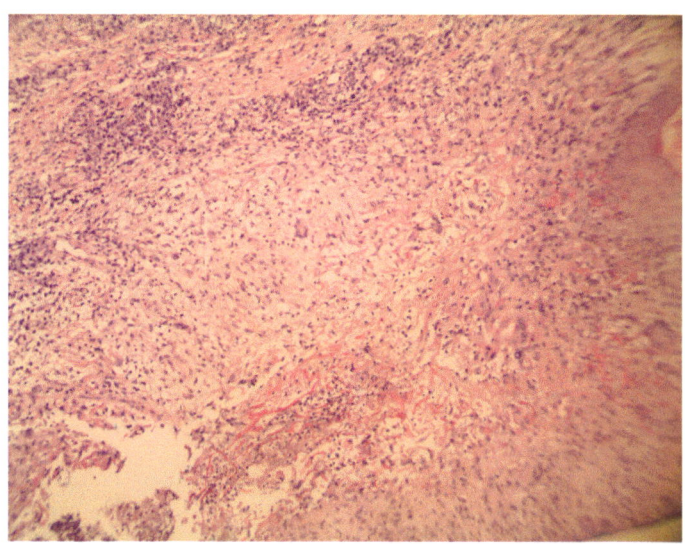

Figure 27.1 H&E 100×, Coccidiodomycosis, inflammation with scattered multinucleated giant cells

Pregnant women who are infected are more likely to present with erythema multiforme or erythema nodosum-like lesions.

Pathology

Coccidioidomycosis lives in the soil where it exists in the mycelial phase with barrel-shaped hyphae. When inhaled, these spores travel into the lungs and become lodged in the alveoli. The host tissue responds with a granulomatous reaction that manifests as caseous necrosis (Fig. 27.1).

Coccidioidomycosis does not affect all ethnicities equally. Those of African, Filipino, Mexican or Native American heritage are more likely to contract the disease. Those of African descent are more likely to develop bone involvement of the disease and Filipinos are more prone to develop fungal meningitis. The reason for this predisposition is still unknown. The majority of infected individuals, approximately 60 %, are

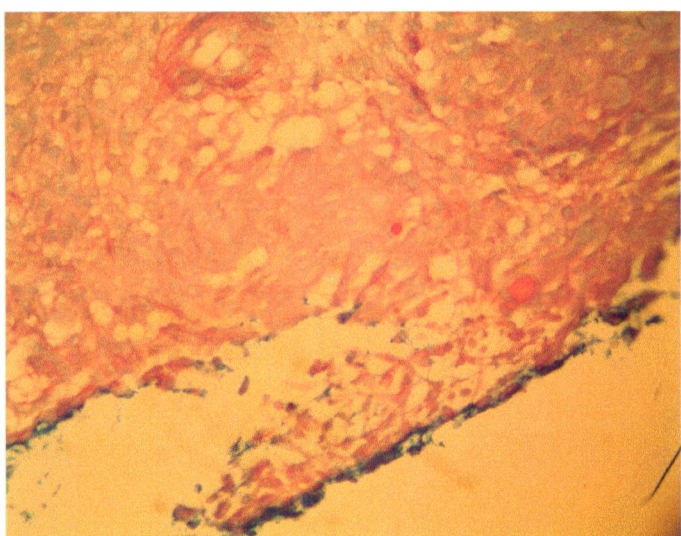

FIGURE 27.2 PAS 1,000×, Along the edge of the tissue, the section shows two endospores

either asymptomatic or present with nonspecific symptoms similar to an upper respiratory infection. In these cases, spontaneous remission may occur within 2 weeks with complete recovery. The remaining 40 % of people will develop cough, night sweats, lethargy, anorexia and arthralgia that is referred to as "desert rheumatism." Disseminated disease involves the bones, skin, and meninges. Coccidioidomycosis tends to occur in individuals with occupations that require field labor like construction workers and farmers.

The diagnosis of coccidioidomycosis can be made using histopathology, culture, serology and imaging studies. Under the microscope, coccidioidomycosis appears as a large spherule filled with endospores that are highlighted with either PAS or silver staining (Fig. 27.2). Cultures of pus, bronchoalveolar sputum (Figs. 27.3 and 27.4), and synovial fluid provide the best results but are dependent on the extent of dissemination. Cultures of blood, pleural fluid, and cerebral spinal fluid can be used but are generally less sensitive.

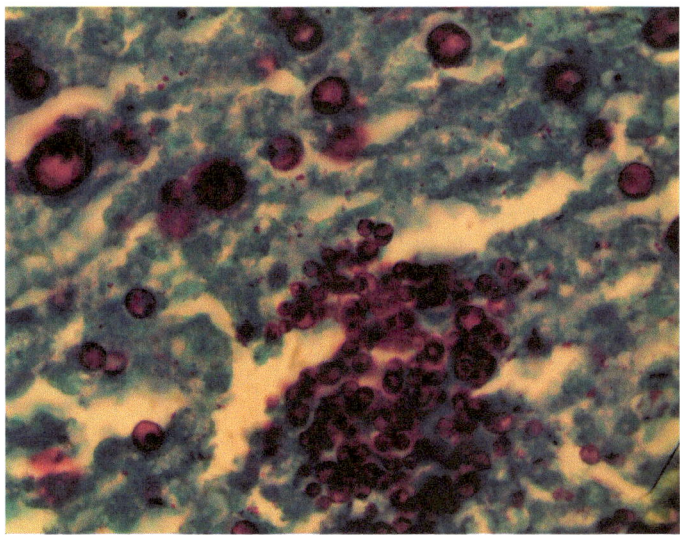

FIGURE 27.3 PAS stain 1,000×, Cocciidiodomycosis shows numerous spores in the lung

Serology is performed to check for elevated serum complement-fixing antibody (CFA) titers. Titers greater than 1:32 indicate disseminated disease. In cases of meningitis, the serology CFA will be low in the blood but positive in the cerebral spinal fluid. Enzyme-linked immunosorbent assay (ELISA) is used to tag 33-kDa antigens and monitor for disease progression and response to treatment. Chest radiography is used to screen for pulmonary disease and may demonstrate hilar adenopathy, pleural effusion, infiltrates, and thin-walled cavities that remain after primary infection.

Treatment Options

The type of medication and duration of treatment is dependent on the location of the infection, the extent, and the immune status of the host. For infections that are deep-seated or meningeal, fluconazole 400 mg to 1.2 g a day is commonly

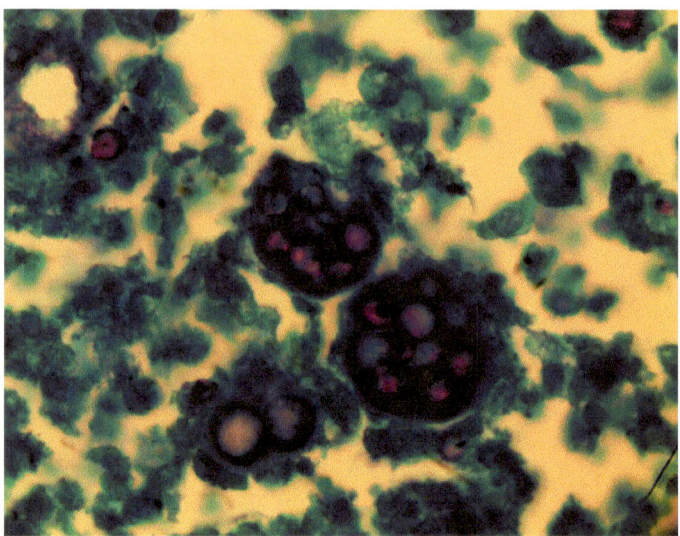

FIGURE 27.4 PAS stain 1,000×, Coccidiodomycosis, endospores are seen within the sporangia

used and is recommended as the first choice for patients with AIDS. Itraconazole 400–600 mg daily is used for patients with joint, bone, lymphatic or genitourinary involvement. Amphotericin B 0.6–1 mg/kg/day for the initial week of therapy and then 0.8 mg/kg every other day until remission is achieved which usually about 1 year. Individuals with meningeal disease are treated for life to prevent reactivation of the disease. In these cases fluconazole 400–1,000 mg daily is recommended indefinitely.

Prevention

Physicians must maintain a high level of suspicion for patients who are natives of travelers to endemic regions. Lab personnel must be warned ahead of time if cultures are sent because aerosolized spores are highly infective.

Recommended Reading

Bennett JE, Dolin R. Coccidioidomycosis. By Mandell GL. 7th ed. N.p.: Waltham, MA: Elsevier Limited; 2010. p. 3333–44.

Brinster NK, Liu V, Diwan AH, McKee PH. Dermatopathology: high-yield pathology. N.p.: Philadelphia, PA: Saunders; 2011.

DiCaudo DJ. Coccidioidomycosis: a review and update. J Am Acad Dermatol. 2006;55(6):929–42.

Ferri FF, Van Dunin D, Opal S, Mylonakis EE. Ferri's Clinical Advisor. N.p.: St Louis, MO: Mosby; 2014.

Galgiani JN, Ampel NM, Blair JE, et al. Coccidioidomycosis. Clin Infect Dis. 2005;41(9):1217–23.

Heymann WR, John BJ, Ian C. "Coccidioidomycosis." Treatment of skin disease: comprehensive therapeutic strategies. By Lebwohl MG. 4th ed. N.p.: Waltham, MA: Elsevier Limited, n.d. 2013;147–49.

Parish JM, Blair JE. Coccidioidomycosis. Mayo Clin Proc. 2008; 83(3):343–48.

Case 28
78 Year Old Brazilian Male with Multiple Skin and Nasal Mucosal Ulcerations

William Eng and Lisa M. Diaz

Clinical and History

A 78 year old male from Brazil presented with a complaint of multiple ulcerations involving the skin and nasal mucosa.

Clinical Differential Diagnosis

- Blastomycosis
- Metastatic malignancy
- Syphilis
- Leishmania

W. Eng, MD (✉)
Department of Pathology, University of Central Florida Medical School, Orlando, FL, USA
e-mail: drwilliameng@yahoo.com

L.M. Diaz, DO
College of Osteopathic Medicine, Lake Erie College of Osteopathic Medicine, Bradenton, FL, USA

R.A. Norman, W. Eng (eds.), *Clinical Cases in Infections and Infestations of the Skin*, Clinical Cases in Dermatology 6, DOI 10.1007/978-3-319-14295-1_28,
© Springer International Publishing Switzerland 2015

Diagnosis

PARACOCCIDIOIDMYCOCOSIS or South American Blastomycosis, is a chronic, progressive systemic mycosis that is caused by the fungus Paracoccidioides brasiliensis. The fungus lives in the soil in endemic regions where it is the leading cause of death in those infected with systemic mycoses. Cases have been reported in all Latin American countries except Chile and those in the Caribbean islands. Eighty percent of reported cases originate from Brazil with the majority occurring in the Sao Paulo state. This infection is seen mostly in men who work outside in rural, agricultural occupations. Risk factors include immunosuppression and a history of smoking.

The clinical appearance of the infection is dependent on the immune status of the host as well as the duration of time that the infection has been present. The classic mucocutaneous lesions of paracoccidioidomycosis are superficial ulcers or strawberry-red granulomas with hemorrhagic punctate spots on the oral mucosa that are referred to as "mulberry-like stomatitis." These nasal and oral lesions may be tender or painful and oral involvement may lead to macrocheilia. Scarring is frequently seen. Involvement of the lungs and larynx result in chronic obstructive pulmonary disease and dysphonia, respectively. Lymphadenopathy is frequently observed, especially in affected individuals younger than 30. The supraclavicular and lymph nodes located in the head are the most commonly affected. They are painfully enlarged and may become suppurative. There are four possible clinical presentations for paracoccidioidomycosis: pulmonary, lymphatic, mucocutaneous or mixed.

Pathology

The fungus is inhaled and then travels to the lungs where it resides. It typically has a 1–3 week incubation period. Eventually it may disseminate to other organs, usually the skin

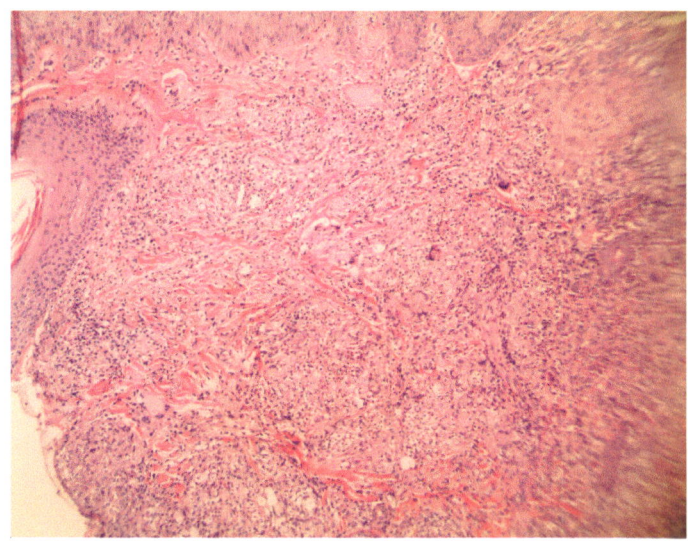

FIGURE 28.1 H&E 100× paracoccidiomycosis, a dense infiltrate of histocytes

and mucous membranes. There are rare reports of direct inoculation and most of these cases occur when individuals brush their teeth with infected twigs, a practice that is observed in rural areas of Brazil. Paracoccidioides brasiliensis is a dimorphic fungus that grows in its mycelial form at room temperature and as yeast in vitro. Interestingly, women are less likely to become infected as the hormone estradiol prevents the conversion of the fungus to its infective yeast form. Its characteristic appearance is akin to a ship's wheel with a central, large thick-walled spherule and multiple narrow-based buds that are organized like the spokes on a wheel.

Diagnosis

The diagnosis can be made histologically by skin biopsy. Periodic acid-Schiff staining reveals yeast with multiple narrow based buds described as a "Mariner's wheel." (Figs. 28.1 and 28.2).

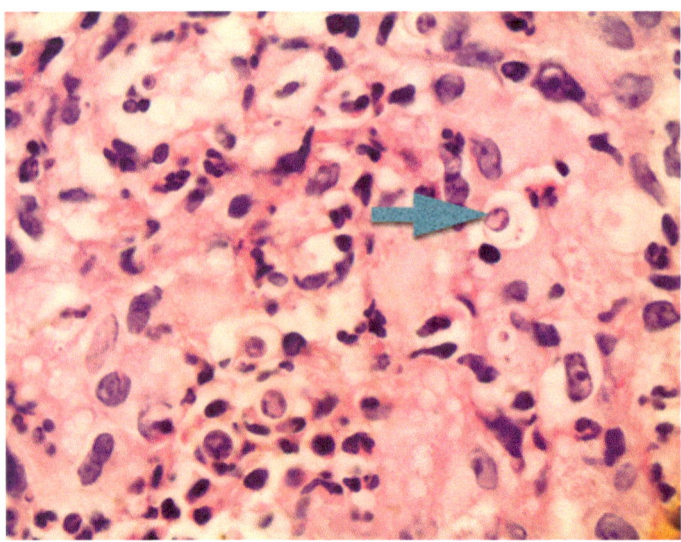

FIGURE 28.2 H&E 1,000×, note central yeast-like organisms with small daughter yeasts at the peripheral rim

Direct examination with a KOH scraping may reveal oval cells in groups or chains. A fungal culture using Sabouraud agar is always recommended however it has low sensitivity and takes 20–30 days to produce growth.

Serological tests are available but not used as they are rarely diagnostic. HIV testing may be performed in patients suspected of infection. Chest radiography should always be performed to check for pulmonary involvement.

Treatment

The first line treatment for moderate cases of infection is itra-conazole 100 mg daily for 6 months If that therapy fails, keto-conazole 400 mg daily for 6–18 months may be used. In severe cases of infection or in cases with meningeal involvement, IV amphotericin B 0.4–0.5 mg/kg is recommended daily until a total dose of 1.5–2.5 mg/kg has been administered.

Prevention

When traveling, it is recommended that endemic regions be avoided. Disease presentation can be delayed with cases reported 60 days after initial infection. Early detection and diagnosis is important to prevent disseminated disease, permanent disfigurement and death. Whenever the combination of pulmonary, cutaneous, mucosal, and lymphatic involvement is observed, paracoccidioidomycosis should be at the top of the differential diagnoses list.

Recommended Reading

Bellissimo-Rodrigues F, Machado AA, Martinez R. Paracocci-dioidomycosis epidemiological features of a 1,000-cases series from a hyperendemic area on the southeast of Brazil. Am J Trop Med Hyg. 2011;85(3):546–50.

Heymann WR, John BJ, Ian C. "Paracoccidioidomycosis." Treatment of skin disease: comprehensive therapeutic strategies. By Lebwohl MG. 4th ed. N.p.: Waltham, MA: Elsevier Limited; 2014. p. 535–38.

Marques SA. Paracoccidioidomycosis. Clin Dermatol. 2012;30(6): 610–5.

Martino-Ortiz BD, Rodriguez-Oviedo ML, Rodriguez-Masi M. Chronic multifocal paracoccidioidomycosis in an immunocompetent adult. Actas Derm-Sifiliograficas. 2012;103(7):645–6.

Menezes VM, Soares BG, Fontes CJ. Drugs for treating paracoccidioidomycosis. Cochrane Database Syst Rev. 2006;(19):CD004967.

Naranjo MS, Trujillo M, Munera MI, Restrepo P, Gomez I, Restrepo A. Treatment of paracoccidioidomycosis with itraconazole. J Med Vet Mycol. 1990;28:67–76.

Ramos-E-Silva M, Saraiva Ldo E. Paracoccidioidomycosis. Dermatol Clin. 2008;26:257–69.

Yasuda MA. Pharmacological management of paracoccidioidomycosis. Expert Opin Pharmacother. 2005;6:385–97.

Case 29
50 Year Old Male with Dark Red Rash Inside Mouth and Left Axillae

William Eng and Martin J. Walsh

Clinical

A 50 year old slightly obese HIV+ male presented with a rash on his left axillae and in his mouth.

Physical Examination

In the oral cavity, the lesion started as a discrete white patch that become progressively confluent (Fig. 29.1). At the groin, the lesions appeared as erythematous, eroded pustular papules that coalesced into "beefy red" plaques (Fig. 29.2). Occasional satellite pustules were seen at the periphery.

W. Eng, MD (✉)
Department of Pathology, University of Central Florida Medical School, Orlando, FL, USA
e-mail: drwilliameng@yahoo.com

M.J. Walsh, MS, BA
Graduate Studies, USF College of Medicine,
Tampa, FL, USA

R.A. Norman, W. Eng (eds.), *Clinical Cases in Infections and Infestations of the Skin*, Clinical Cases in Dermatology 6, DOI 10.1007/978-3-319-14295-1_29,
© Springer International Publishing Switzerland 2015

161

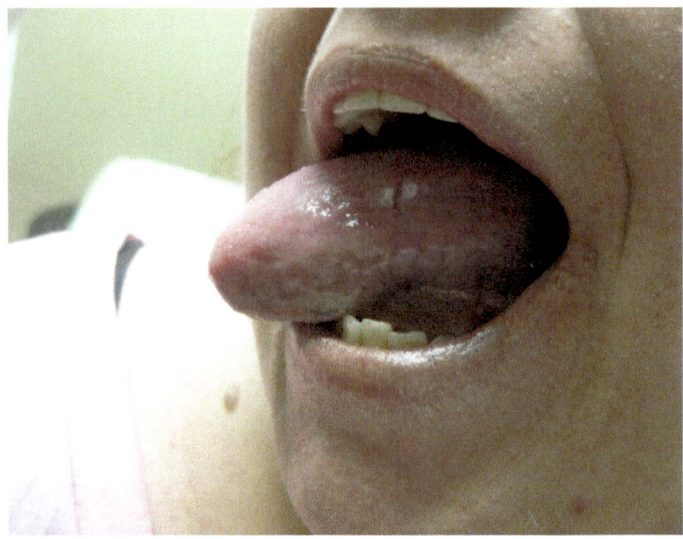

FIGURE 29.1 Candidiasis, whitish material attached to the tongue (thrush)

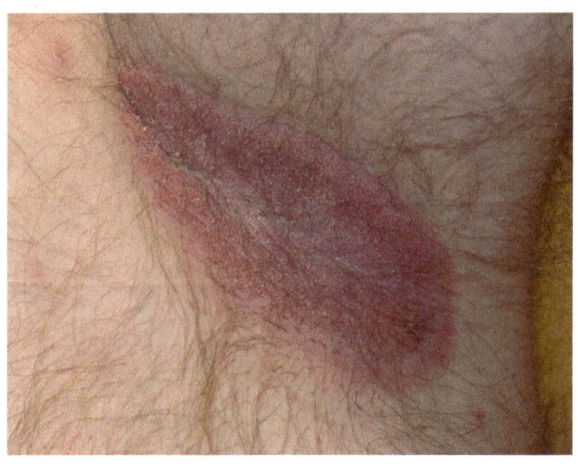

FIGURE 29.2 Candidiasis, beefy red plaque at the axillae

Clinical Differential Diagnosis

(Skin Fold Rash)

- Intertrigo
- Tinea
- Psoriasis
- Erythrasma
- Seborrheic dermatitis
- Candidiasis

Histopathology

The changes of an infection can include an irregular psoriasi-form hyperplasia with an overlying serum crust with neutro-phils. The dermis shows a mixed infiltrate of histiocytes, lymphocytes, plasma cells, and occasional giant cell. The PAS stain shows yeasts (Fig. 29.3).

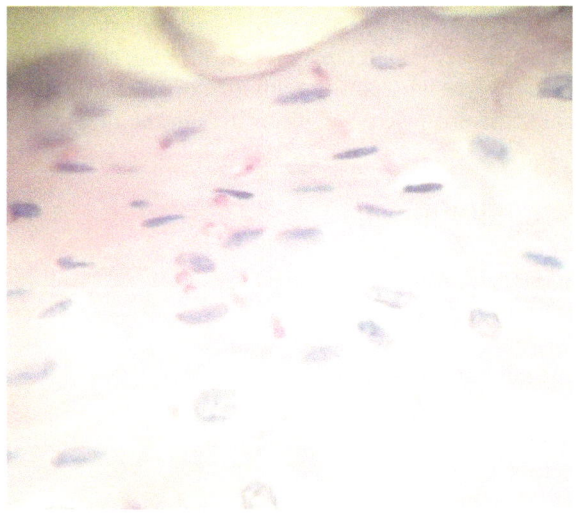

FIGURE 29.3 PAS stain 400×, Candidiasis, *pink-red* yeasts and pseu-dohyphae

Diagnosis

CANDIDIASIS (yeast) infections encompasses over 200 species. It's appearance can vary from yeast to hyphae to pseudohyphae forms. Candidia albicans is the most common pathogen which can affect any body site. Colonization of the oral cavity is common in up to 50 % of individuals, but it acts pathogenic in immunocompromised (HIV infected) individuals. In the groin area, moist and warm environments due to obesity, occlusive clothing, and diabetes contributes to candidiasis infection. Other factors such as mechanical, nutritional, mediations, and systemic illnesses can contribute to a higher risk factor of developing an infection. It can be identified on tissue sections by PAS, GMS or by other fungal stains as budding yeast structures.

The pattern of inflammation which mirrors the opposite side of the skin can be caused by various infections bacterial (erythrasma), yeast (candidiasis, seborrheic dermatitis), fungal (tinea cruris). In infants, this (diaper) pattern may be a secondary reaction to persistent irritant and moisture (urine-soaked diaper). Psoriasis at the groin area appears without the typical overlying parakeratosis scales although the underlying sharply demarcated erythematous base remains present (inverse psoriasis). Routine microscopic examination and special stains for microorganisms aids in the diagnosis.

Treatment Options

- Fluconazole- systemic
- Nystatin- oral
- Clotrimazole troches- oral
- Topical imidazole- vulvovaginitis
- Clotrimazole- skin
- Econazole- skin
- Ciclopirox – skin
- Miconazole- skin
- Ketoconazole – skin
- Nystatin – skin

Recommended Reading

Goldsmith LA et al. Fitzpatrick's dermatology in general medicine. 8th ed. New York: McGraw-Hill Co; 2012. p. 2298–06.

Part IV
Infestations

Case 30
45 Year Old Male with Multiple Open Sores After Returning from South American Jungle

William Eng and Lisa M. Diaz

Clinical and History

A 45 year old white male recently developed multiple open sores after returning from visiting the South America jungle. He reported being bitten by multiple insects.

Physical Examination

The skin showed multiple scattered ulcerations of various sizes

W. Eng, MD (✉)
Department of Pathology, University of Central Florida Medical School, Orlando, FL, USA
e-mail: drwilliameng@yahoo.com

L.M. Diaz, DO
College of Osteopathic Medicine, Lake Erie College of Osteopathic Medicine, Bradenton, FL, USA

R.A. Norman, W. Eng (eds.), *Clinical Cases in Infections and Infestations of the Skin*, Clinical Cases in Dermatology 6, DOI 10.1007/978-3-319-14295-1_30,
© Springer International Publishing Switzerland 2015

Clinical Differential Diagnosis

- Insect bite
- Leishmania
- Lymphoma
- Metastatic carcinoma

Histopathology

These protozoa are dimorphic organisms that take the form of a flagellated promastigote within the sandfly vector but then transform into an a flegellated amastigote within the host. The protozoa migrate from the gut of the sandfly to the mouth and then are transmitted to the host when the sandfly takes a blood meal. The protozoa is engulfed by host macrophages and is then transferred to phagolysosomes where it resides and replicates until the cell ruptures and spreads to infect other macrophages.

Each clinical form of leishmania has its own distinct appearance under the microscope. Localized cutaneous leishmania demonstrates granulomatous inflammation in the dermis and epidermis. Diffuse cutaneous leishmania shows amastigotes within macrophages. Mucosal leishmania demonstrates destruction of tissue including any nearby bone or cartilage. Visceral leishmania shows cell hyperplasia in the reticuloendothelial organs including the spleen, liver, and lymph nodes with amastigotes present.

Diagnosis

Leishmania is an umbrella term for a clinical spectrum of diseases caused by intracellular protozoa that are transmitted by phlebotomine sandflies. The protozoa responsible for causing leishmaniasis in humans fall under two subgenera: Leishmania and Viannia. Leishmaniasis may affect the skin, mucosal surfaces or reticuloendothelial visceral organs. The cutaneous manifestation of leishmaniasis typically has a benign course, however, it may lead to disfigurement if treatment is delayed. Mucosal and visceral organ involvement indicates a more dangerous affliction with a disease course that may lead to increased morbidity and mortality.

Leishmaniasis is estimated to affect 10–50 million people in endemic tropical and subtropical regions worldwide. There are reported cases in all continents except for Australia and Antarctica. Leishmaniasis is divided into four distinct clinical forms, each with its own individual cause, reservoir, endemic region, and clinical manifestation. These forms are listed in order of increasing severity: localized cutaneous, diffuse cutaneous, mucosal, and visceral. For simplicity and clarity, each of these forms will be discussed individually.

Localized cutaneous leishmania, also referred to as oriental sore, is a non-tender shallow ulcer with raised erythematous and indurated margins that occurs at the site of a sandfly bite. There may be one or several lesions present that usually begin as papules on exposed skin, usually on the face and arms. Over time, these papules enlarge and ulcerate. A brisk granulomatous reaction is found in the dermis and scattered multi-nucleated giant cells and macrophages filled with organisms (Fig. 30.1). At high magnification, the organisms are seen by routine H&E staining as oval organisms with a kinetoplast (dark spot) at the edge (Fig. 30.2). Those that are caused by *L. major* and *L. mexicana* typically heal on their own within 6 months of presentation leaving behind a scar. The Viannia subgroup tends to cause lesions that are larger and more chronic in nature. In addition, this subgroup is more likely to present with sporotrichoid streaking and regional lymphadenopathy.

Diffuse cutaneous leishmania is rare and is caused by *L. mexicana* and *L. aethiopica* in certain endemic regions. Unlike localized cutaneous leishmaniasis, these lesions are large and often widespread on the body. They may present as nonulcerating macules, papules, nodules or plaques. Similar to localized cutaneous leishmaniasis, these lesions initially present on exposed surfaces like the face and arms but then disseminated widely over the course of several years.

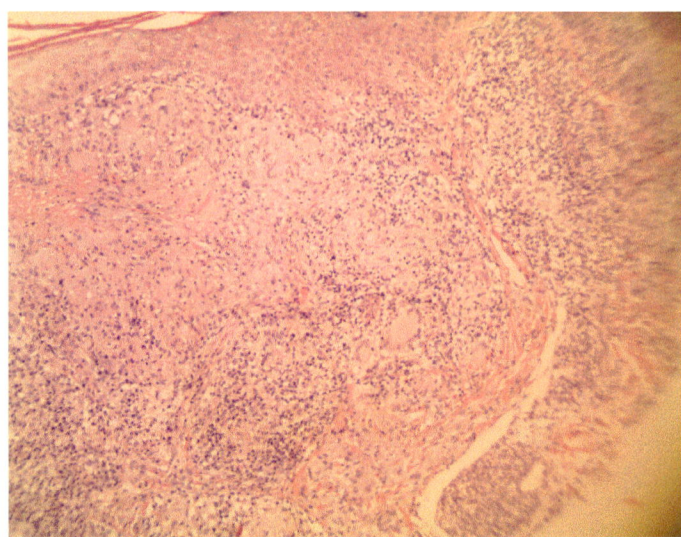

FIGURE 30.1 H&E 100×, Leishmania, a mixed inflammatory infiltrate with scattered multi-nucleated

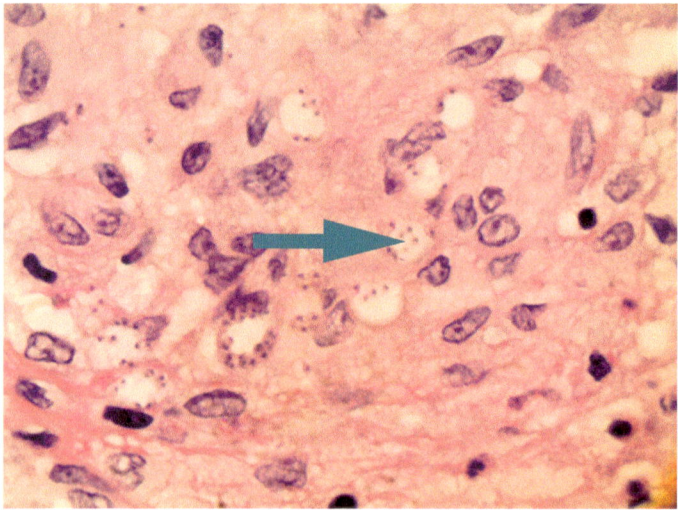

FIGURE 30.2 H&E 1,000×, Leishmania, small clusters of organisms between the histiocytes

Muscosal leishmania is a more serious form of leishmaniasis that is usually caused by the Viannia subgenera. This uncommon presentation is caused by hematogenous spread from a cutaneous lesion to the nasopharyngeal mucosa. In the majority of cases, it occurs in individuals who have had a cutaneous lesion within the previous 2 years. However, there are reports of it occurring years after the primary lesion had resolved. Those affected tend to suffer from nasal congestion, epistaxis, and edema. If left untreated, it can cause destruction of the nose and mouth leading to severe disfigurement.

Visceral leishmania, also known as kala-azar, is the most serious clinical form of the disease. In the New World and the Mediterranean regions children less than 5 years old are most commonly affected and *L. infantum* and *L. chagasi* are responsible. In Africa and Asia older children and adults are more likely to be infected and the causative organism is *L. donovani*. Approximately 25 % of the infected individuals will develop the characteristic symptoms of hepatosplenomegaly, high fever, and cachexia within 6 months of contracting the disease. If the individual is untreated, the disease progresses with pancytopenia and severe anemia that may lead to heart failure. Ultimately, the cause of death is a result of secondary bacterial infection and occurs in more than 90 % of the untreated population.

There is a skin complication known as post kala-azar dermal leishmaniasis that presents in some patients who were treated in the past for visceral leishmania. They characteristically begin around the mouth and spread over the face and torso. These lesions appear as erythematous or hypopigmented macules, papules or nodules. It is seen most commonly in India and Sudan and the causative organism is *L. donovani*.

The microscopic diagnosis can be made by visualization of the kinetoplast, which has a characteristic appearance under oil-immersion microscopy. Thin smears of tissue under light microscopy examination, biopsy of lymph nodes or Giemsa-stained tissue sections may all be used to demonstrate the presence of amastigotes. Tissue culture or polymerase chain reaction with demonstration of parasite DNA may also be used. An enzyme-linked immunosorbent assay (ELISA) using K39, a recombinant antigen, is highly sensitive for visceral leishmania.

A scattered pattern of lesions with ulceration brings up the differential of infection and malignancy. Microscopic examination along with special stains can aid in distinguishing what type of infection and malignancy is present.

Treatment Options

Anti-leishmanial treatment is only recommended in cases that do not heal spontaneously within 3–4 months, those with lymphatic involvement, or in those cases that may result in permanent disfigurement or disability. It is not recommended in all cases because there is a high rate of spontaneous resolution without any medical intervention. Every patient that is diagnosed with visceral or mucosal leishmania is automatically treated.

Sodium stibogluconate has been used successfully for leishmania treatment for decades. In cases of localized or diffuse cutaneous involvement, 20 mg/kg/day IV or IM is recommended for 20 days. In cases of mucosal or visceral leishmania the same medication is recommended for an additional 8 days. It is not unusual for patients to require multiple treatments in cases of extensive disease. In the past, cure rates with this treatment varied from 50 to 100 %. However, certain regions are reporting resistance to this medication. In these cases, amphotericin B 0.5–1.0 mg/kg daily up to 20 days is recommended. Other medications used successfully include: paromomycin, recombinant human interferon gamma, miltefosine, ketoconazole, and fluconazole.

Prevention

In areas of high risk insect repellent that contains DEET, proper protective clothing, and fly nets are strongly encouraged. The practice of "Leishmanization" is still utilized in some endemic regions. In this practice, mothers expose the buttocks of their young children to sandflies so that the cutaneous lesions and scars will develop in a covered area as opposed to somewhere more visible like the face or arms. Ultimately, early diagnosis and treatment in severe cases of disease are essential.

Recommended Reading

Bennett JE, Dolin R. Leishmania Species. In: Mandell GL, editor. Principles and practice of infectious diseases. 7th ed. N.p.: Waltham, MA: Elsevier; 2010. p. 3463–80.

Stanton BF, St. Geme JW, Schor NF, Behrman RE. Leishmaniasis. In: Kliegman RM, editor. Nelson textbook of pediatrics. 19th ed. N.p.: Waltham, MA: Elsevier; 2011. 1186–90.

Zijlstra EE, Musa AM, Khalil EA, et al. Post-kala-azar dermal leishmaniasis. Lancet Infect Dis. 2003;3(2):87–98.

Case 31
67 Year Old with Slight Erythema of the Nose

William Eng and Martin J. Walsh

History and Clinical

A 67-year-old female presented with a request for a full body examination. The patient has had a history of allergies including, iodine, sulfa medications, and Fluphenazine.

Physical Examination

The patient's nose showed a flesh colored papule with a slightly dilated follicular orifice on the left side (Fig. 31.1).

W. Eng, MD (✉)
Department of Pathology, University of Central Florida Medical School, Orlando, FL, USA
e-mail: drwilliameng@yahoo.com

M.J. Walsh, MS, BA
Graduate Studies, USF College of Medicine, Tampa, FL, USA

R.A. Norman, W. Eng (eds.), *Clinical Cases in Infections and Infestations of the Skin*, Clinical Cases in Dermatology 6, DOI 10.1007/978-3-319-14295-1_31,
© Springer International Publishing Switzerland 2015

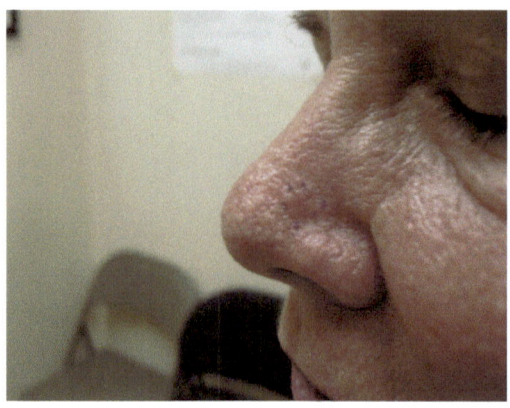

FIGURE 31.1 Demodex mite. A circular lesion marked by ink dots was biopsied

Clinical Differential Diagnosis

- Fibrous papule
- Basal cell carcinoma
- Sebaceous hyperplasia
- Cyst
- Demodex folliculitis

Histopathology

Sections showed a portion of an insect within the follicular infundibulum. A mild perifollicular of lymphocytes and histiocytes were found (Fig. 31.2).

Diagnosis

DEMODEX FOLLICULITIS. Two mites, Demodex folliculorum hominis and brevis, typically reside on the face, particularly on the nose. There is debate whether these mites are the cause of rosacea, perioral dermatitis, and suppurative folliculitis.

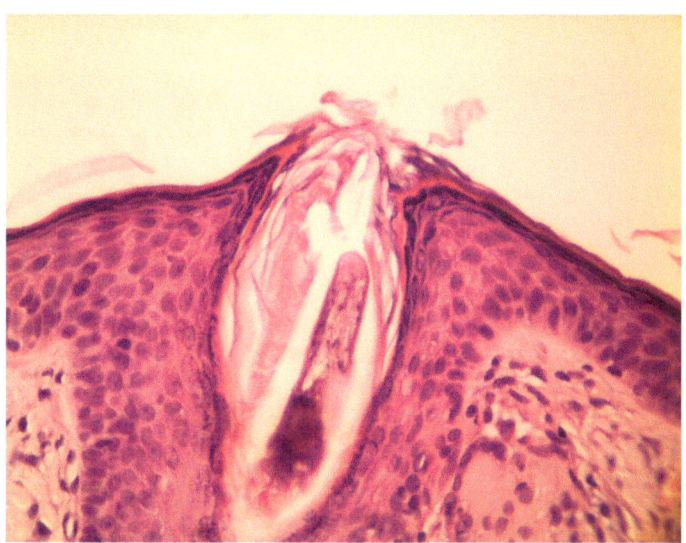

FIGURE 31.2 H&E 100×, Demodex mite, note the multi-nucleated giant cell to the right of the follicular epithelium

A fibrous papule shows telangiectasis with a fibrotic stroma. Basal cell carcinoma produces nests of hyperchromatic cells in the dermis. Sebaceous hyperplasia shows enlarged sebaceous lobules without cytologic atypia. Cysts are lined with squamous, apocrine, or eccrine cells.

Treatment

Since most dermatologist consider this incidental finding not a disease state.

Recommended Reading

1. Goldsmith LA et al. Fitzpatrick's dermatology in general medicine. 8th ed. New York: McGraw-Hill Co; 2012. p. 2572.

Case 32
57 Year Old Male with Multiple Widespread Excoriations

William Eng and Martin J. Walsh

History and Clinical

An 57-year-old male presented with a rash on his left proximal upper arm and upper chest. Around seven discrete lesions were found on the upper left back and about four were found on the right upper back which worsen at night. Also lesions were found on the proximal thigh. The patient also exhibited pruritus His medical history consisted of a fracture of the radial bone, diverticulitis, depression, hypertension, viral hepatitis, dementia, dysphagia, anemia, encephalopathy, subdural hemorrhage, muscle weakness, chronic respiratory failure, and seborrheic dermatitis on the scalp. There was a previous treatment for scabies with elimite and stromectol.

W. Eng, MD (✉)
Department of Pathology, University of Central Florida Medical School, Orlando, FL, USA
e-mail: drwilliameng@yahoo.com

M.J. Walsh, MS, BA
Graduate Studies, USF College of Medicine, Tampa, FL, USA

R.A. Norman, W. Eng (eds.), *Clinical Cases in Infections and Infestations of the Skin*, Clinical Cases in Dermatology 6, DOI 10.1007/978-3-319-14295-1_32, © Springer International Publishing Switzerland 2015

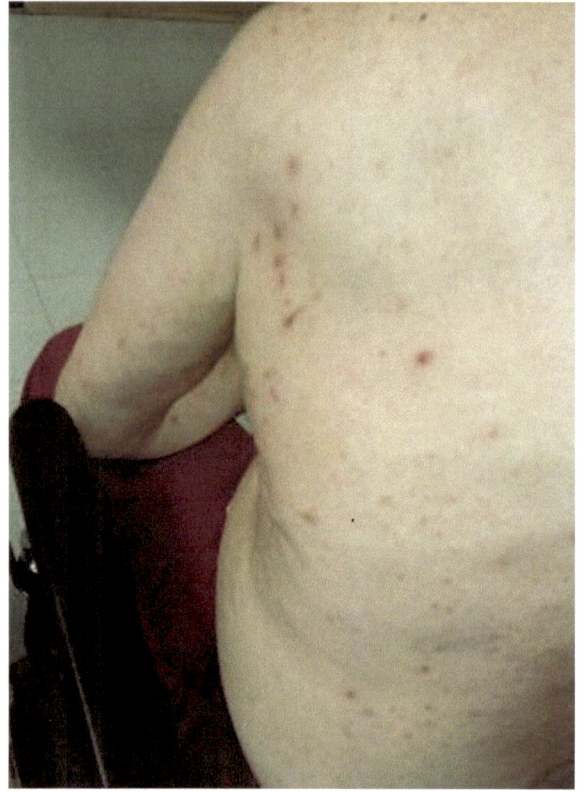

FIGURE 32.1 Scabies, extremely pruritic papules in a widespread pattern

Physical Examination

The patient exhibited multiple reddish, brown, poorly defined macules with a dry, adherent scaly appearance (Fig. 32.1) His complete blood count (CBC) showed an increased percentage of eosinophils (9.2 %) and (10.2 %) on a repeated CBC.

Clinical Differential Diagnosis

- Drug eruption
- Scabies

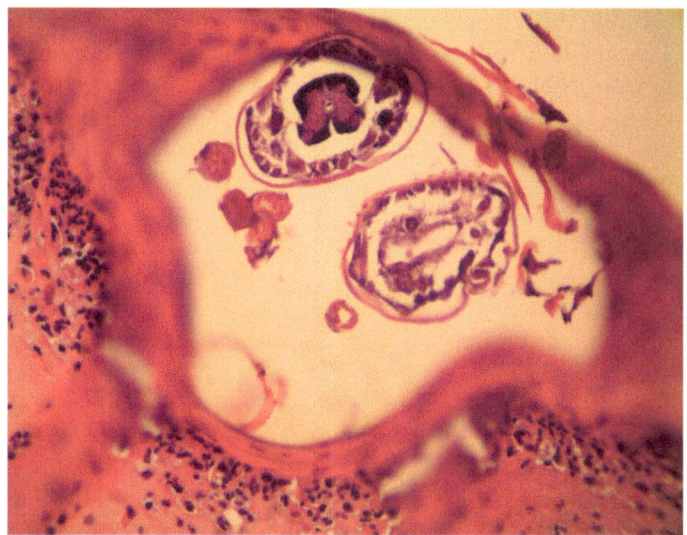

FIGURE 32.2 H&E 400× Scabies mite cross-section of mite within a burrow

- Bedbugs
- Atopic dermatitis
- Contact dermatitis
- Urticaria stage of bullous pemphigoid

Histopathology

The first biopsy was from the trunk which showed spongiotic dermatitis, but no insect body was seen. A second biopsy was taken which showed features of an insect bite, and negative results for fungus in the Periodic Acid-Schiff stain. A third biopsy was taken from the trunk and extremities which did show an insect residing within the cornified layer (Fig. 32.2).

Diagnosis

SCABIES (Sarcoptes scabies var. homini). This infestation occurs worldwide affecting all ages, races, and socioeconomic levels. A typical host can harbor 3–50 insects, but those who are immunocompromised can have millions of mites. Transmission is most commonly through personal contact, however, sharing of objects/clothes is also a mode of transmission particularly in children. It is not uncommon infestation in areas of poor hygiene with increased concentrations of people, i.e., nursing homes, prisons, dormitories. Although medications are effective, patients are often re-infected if their environment has not been properly sanitized or by a non-treated individual. The mite's entire life cycle is completely on human skin. The female mite will burrow through the stratum corneum at a rate of 1 cm/day during which time, they will lay one to three eggs. The eggs hatch into larva 10 days after which they mature on the skin surface. This activity continues till the end of their 30 day life cycle. The mites can live up to 3 days off the skin. Common sites of infestation include the finger webs, wrist, lateral palms, elbows, axillae, scrotum, penis, labia, and areolae. The hyperkeratotic plaques (Norwegian scabies) which represents extensive infestation can develop in the physically and mentally disabled, as well as those who have epidermolysis bullosa and neurosensory impairment.

The symptoms of intense itching can bring up the possibility of a drug eruption. Correlation with drug intake history would be helpful. Microscopically, a drug eruption presents with a perivascular lymphocytic infiltrate with eosinophils. This may be similar to an allergic contact dermatitis and atopic dermatitis. Bed bug bites often occur at night and patients typically notice blood spots on their sheets.

Treatment Options

- Permethrin 5 % cream
- Lindane 1 % lotion
- Crotamiton 10 % cream
- Precipitated sulfur
- Benzyl Benzoate 10 % lotion
- Ivermectin 200 ug/kg

Recommended Reading

1. Goldsmith LA et al. Fitzpatrick's dermatology in general medicine. 8th ed. New York: McGraw-Hill Co; 2012. p. 2569–72.

Case 33
53 Year Old Female with Multiple Areas of Erythema on Scalp

William Eng and Martin J. Walsh

History and Clinical

An 53-year-old female presented with an erythematous area on her scalp. The patient also presented with chronic pruritus on her right lower extremity. She was a new patient that was living in a local assisted living facility.

Physical Examination

The patient revealed localized and circumscribed thick skin area with lichenification on her right lower extremity as well as erythematous eruptions in the localized region. On the scalp, the erythematous area also showed semi-translucent material attached to the hair shaft (Fig. 33.1).

W. Eng, MD (✉)
Department of Pathology, University of Central Florida Medical School, Orlando, FL, USA
e-mail: drwilliameng@yahoo.com

M.J. Walsh, MS, BA
Graduate Studies, USF College of Medicine,
Tampa, FL, USA

R.A. Norman, W. Eng (eds.), *Clinical Cases in Infections and Infestations of the Skin*, Clinical Cases in Dermatology 6, DOI 10.1007/978-3-319-14295-1_33,
© Springer International Publishing Switzerland 2015
187

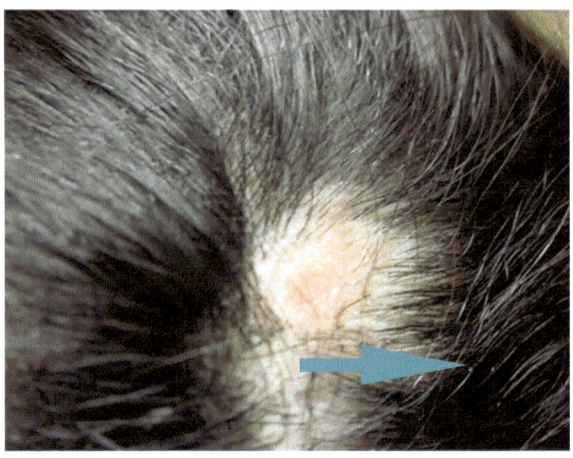

FIGURE 33.1 Head lice

Clinical Differential Diagnosis

Seborrheic dermatitis

- Insect bite
- Pediculosis (Lice)

Eczema

- Psoriasis
- Piedra

Histopathology

Multiple strands of gray hair were removed and submitted for microscopic evaluation. Examination revealed an egg sac attached to the hair shaft (Fig. 33.2).

Diagnosis

PEDICULOSIS (LICE), three types of lice species are identified; Pediculus humans capitis (head lice), Pediculus humans humans (body lice), and Phthirus pubis (pubic/crab lice

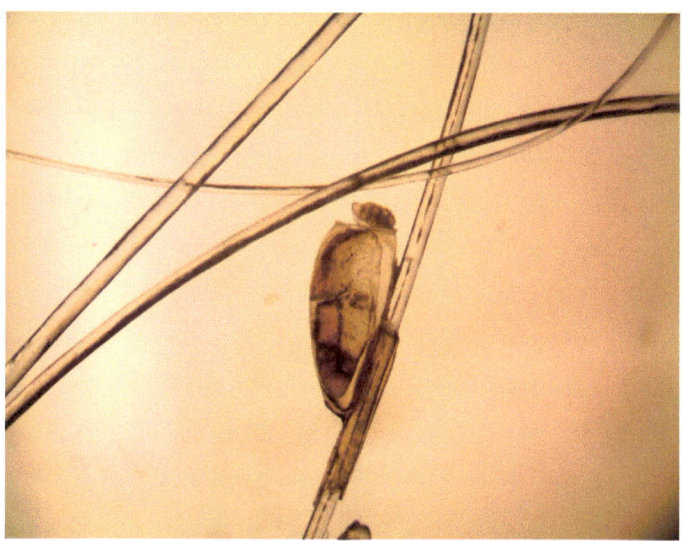

FIGURE 33.2 Unstain, 40×, head lice egg (nit) attached to hair shaft

Fig. 33.1). The infestation is spread by close physical contact and sharing of headgear, combs, brushes, and pillows. However, the incidence is low in blacks due to the inability of the female lice to attach their egg to curly hair. The lice eggs (nits) are easily dislodged which promotes infestation of additional individuals. These insects have three pairs of claw-like legs for grasping hair shafts. Their entire life cycle is spent on the hair where the female lice lays five to ten eggs per day. After 10 days, the eggs hatch and mature in another 14 days. Lice can survive up to 2 days away from the host, while nits can survive up to 10 days. On the scalp, the lice commonly are located on the occipital and retroauricular regions. They survive by blood-sucking the host, thus signs can include an erythematous macule with excoriation and scaling. Diagnosis is made by direct observation of nits on the hair shaft or by locating live lice using a fine comb.

Crab lice is has a shorter length and a wider body than head lice (Fig. 33.3). It also has a shorter lifespan, 3 weeks, but can survive up to 3 days away from the host. The nits also can survive up to 10 days off the body. While sexual transmission

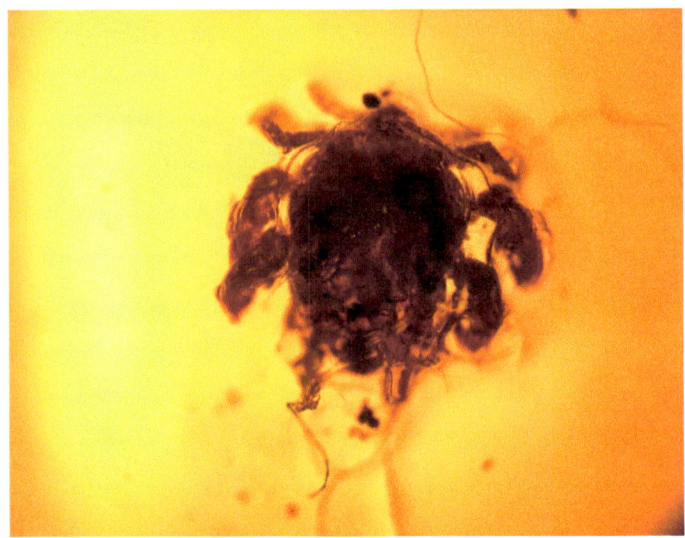

FIGURE 33.3 Unstained 40×, crab lice

of crab lice is the most common of transmission, contact with infected clothing has also been known to be infectious.

The differential of inflammation on the scalp can often be resolved by a punch biopsy. Seborrheic dermatitis which is actually a yeast infection can be identified by the follicular parakeratosis. Psoriasis can appear similar, but there is thinning of the rete ridges with collections of neutrophils (Munro's microabscess). Piedra is a fungal infection of the hair which can produce a dandruff-like condition like psoriasis and seborrheic dermatitis.

Treatment Options

- Physical

  Shaving all hair
  Wet combing
  Cleaning clothing and bedsheets
  Household members

- Permethrin
- Malathion
- Carbaryl
- Lindane
- Invermectin

Recommended Reading

Goldsmith LA et al. Fitzpatrick's dermatology in general medicine. 8th ed. New York: McGraw-Hill Co; 2012. p. 2573–78.

Case 34
6 Year Old White Boy with a Rash on Buttock

William Eng and Robert A. Norman

History and Clinical

The patient is a 6 year old that had been taken to the emergency room and to a pediatrician for a rash and pruritus on the buttocks and was given hydrocortisone cream with no help.

The child has a history of seizure disorders. He had no previous history of the same rash on the buttocks.

The parents stated the child often plays in the dirt along with their dogs and cats.

On examination, a distinct serpiginous and elevated area was noted (see photo) along with several areas of erythema and vesiculation (Fig. 34.1).

W. Eng, MD (✉)
Department of Pathology, University of Central Florida Medical School, Orlando, FL, USA
e-mail: drwilliameng@yahoo.com

R.A. Norman, DO
Medical Director, Dermatology Healthcare,
Tampa, FL, USA

R.A. Norman, W. Eng (eds.), *Clinical Cases in Infections and Infestations of the Skin*, Clinical Cases in Dermatology 6, DOI 10.1007/978-3-319-14295-1_34,
© Springer International Publishing Switzerland 2015

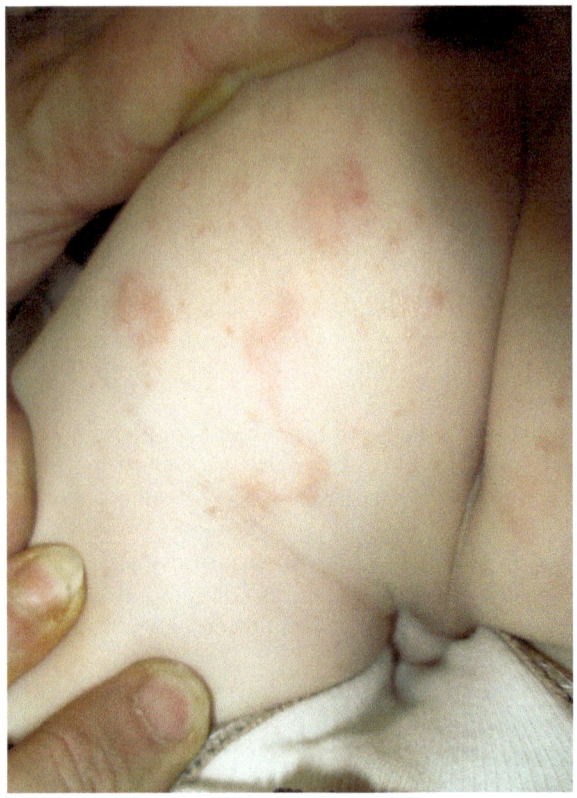

FIGURE 34.1 Cutaneous larva migrans, serpiginous pattern

Differential Diagnosis

Hookworm
Impetigo
Atopic Dermatitis
Cutaneous Larva Migrans

Diagnosis

CUTANEOUS LARVA MIGRANS. The predominantly
cause of human hookworm disease is the nematode parasites
Necator americanus and Ancylostoma duodenale. The

disease is acquired through skin exposure to larvae in soil contaminated by human feces. Atopic dermatitis is usually seen in the antecubital and popliteal areas. Impetigo is often on the face in children and has a distinct crusted pattern.

Cutaneous larva migrans (CLM) is usually confined to the skin of the buttocks, feet or abdomen and is serpiginous and often highly pruritic. When a child such as this patient presents with a rash and with the history of playing in the dirt, it is important to carefully look for the characteristic serpiginous pattern of CLM.

The etiology is dog and cat hookworms who are the normal hosts and, the worm eggs pass through the feces and hatch in moist, warm, sandy soil. The skin irritation is due to a hypersensitivity reaction to the worms (nematodes) and their byproducts.

The disease primarily occurs during warmer months of the year in tropical and subtropical climates. The most common cause of CLM is Ancylostoma braziliense, a dog and cat hookworm found in the United States, Central America, South America, and the Caribbean.

Treatment

Cutaneous larva migrans (CLM) is treated with anthelminthics. Pruritus generally resolves within 24–72 h and serpiginous tracts resolve within 7–10 days. Topical corticosteroids can be used for the relief of pruritus. On occasion oral and topical antibiotic may be used if there is secondary impetiginization or cellulitis.

Index

R.A. Norman, W. Eng (eds.), *Clinical Cases in Infections*
and Infestations of the Skin, Clinical Cases in Dermatology 6,
DOI 10.1007/978-3-319-14295-1,
© Springer International Publishing Switzerland 2015